=:+:=:+:=:+:=:+:=:+:=:+:=:+:=:+:=:+:=:

Meridian Metaphors

Psychology of the Meridians & Major Organs

=:+:=:+:=:+:=:+:=:+:=:+:=:+:=:+:=:+:=:

Bruce Dickson, MSS, MA

InnerSunshine Press

I0475206

To Learn More:

https://HolisticBrainBalance.wordpress.com

Meridian Metaphors; Psychology of the Meridians & Major Organs

Dedicated to expanding the ministry of John-Roger

The thing we are looking for,

is the thing we are looking with.

~ Ernest Holmes, Founder of Religious Science

The future is already here;

it's just not very well distributed yet

~ William Gibson, author, *Neuromancer*

eBook Edition License Notes

Table of Contents

Table of Contents

InnerSunshine Press Book Titles

All titles dedicated to expanding the ministry of John-Roger. These are resources for those looking for self-healing thru self-connection.

Caution ~ Most titles contain exercises require facility with visualizing and/or self-testing with God as your Partner.

Not all images appear in both paper and epub versions. All written with humor by a Waldorf-trained, practicing Health Intuitive.

Best Practices in Group Process Series

Putting healthy group process at the center of thriving, Progressive orgs of all kinds

1) **Heartfelt Facilitators Notebook**; Best Practices Facilitating Large/Small Group Events (2022)

2) **Milling and Dyad Questions** for Learning Conversations in Personal Growth Live Events (2017)

3) **Scripted Closed-Eye-Processes** for Live Personal Growth Event Facilitators and Group Leaders (2017)

New Directions in Holistic Brain Balance

1) **Holistic Neurology;** Connecting with Our Two Nervous Systems, Head-brain and Gut-Brain - Our Two Nervous Systems, Head-spine (cerebral) and enteric (gut), Neurology for purposes of personal growth, the physiological basis for Self-esteem and Self-concept (2nd ed 2023)

2) **Our Four Brain Quadrants**

3) **Reactivity Is Our Best Friend**

4) **Forgive from Your Soul,** Slow-Motion Self-Forgiveness, the Missing Manual

5) **Inner Sunshine** *and How to Make More*; Assessing neurotransmitter production with self-testing; The simple complexity of our unconscious

6) **Practical Epigenetics,** *Best Practices in Belief Change Work,*

7) **Self, Others, World, God**, Our Four Categories of Relationship and Support Support

Best Sellers in Energy Medicine Series

Meridian Metaphors, Psychology of the Meridians and Major Organs - 115 pgs 34,000 words.

The NEW Energy Anatomy: Nine new views of human energy; No clairvoyance required.

Rest of Energy Medicine Series

Reversal of Learning Style at Puberty; How Developing Self-esteem Precedes Self-concept--and Why; Self-confidence Equals Self-esteem Plus Self-concept (99 cent booklet)

Breast Cancer & Over-giving; Therapeutic Metaphors for Women's Issues

Your Symbol of Peace and How to Use It 5,600 words

You have FIVE bodies PACME; Spiritual Geography 101

VAKOG to KAVOG, NLP Senses Updated in Light of the Inner Child 7,032 words

From 5 to 12 Senses, How We Use Multiple Senses to Triangulate, Multiple Intelligences 2.0 10,875 words

How We Heal; and, Why do we get sick? Including 35 more precise Q&A on wellness.

You have FIVE bodies, PACME, Spiritual Geography 101

Self-Healing 101! Seven Experiments in Self-healing, You Can Do at Home to Awaken the Inner Healer, 2nd edition.

Shadow Hero Workbook, Lessons to purify the Hero archetype in you; Healthy vs. Unhealthy Hero behavior; Unconscious Patterns 201

Adequate and Sufficient Psychic Self-protection; For Healers and Energy Medicine Practitioners

Expanding Human Senses from 5 to 12; Rudolf Steiner's 12 Senses to VAKOG to KAVOG

Unconscious Patterns in the Light of the Inner Child and NLP - Our unconscious is highly patterned. You can understand and learn these patterns.

Balance on All Levels PACME+Soul - Finally, a comprehensive holistic theory; and, general holistic experimental method.

Inner Family + Inner Court, The Four Archetypes of Our Gut and Head as internal parts. Expands the work of Paul Dennison, Ned Herrmann, Katherine Benziger and Bertrand Babinet's Babinetics.

Personal Habit Tracking as a Spiritual Exercise - Use self-connection to bridge into your Inner Wisdom

Your Habit Body, An Owner's Manual - Our habits are our best friends; why then, do we make the same errors over and over again?

"**Willingness to heal** is the pre-requisite for all healing"

Radical Cell Wellness—Especially for women! Cell psychology for everyone; A coherent theory of illness and wellness

The Five Puberties, Growing new eyes to see children and developmental age afresh.

The Meaning of Illness is Now an Open Book, Cross-referencing illness and issues

Rudolf Steiner's Fifth Gospel in Story Form The most psychologically astute portrait of JC from Steiner and Emil Bock.

Balance on All Levels PACME+Soul - Finally, a comprehensive holistic theory; and, general holistic experimental method; The Three Sciences we use everyday; Holistic Psychology 2.0. Available as one giant book (paper, eBook), or divided into ten chunks of about equal size, one to four chapters each (eBook only).

Best Practices in Energy Medicine Series

Rudolf Steiner's Fifth Gospel in Story Form - Topics include the TWO Jesus children and the active participation of the Buddha in the Christ event.

Meridian Metaphors, Psychology of the Meridians and Major Organs **-** 115 pgs 34,000 words. A best seller in this series).

The NEW Energy Anatomy: Nine new views of human energy; No clairvoyance required (a best selling title in this series).

Self-Healing 101! Seven Experiments in Self-healing, You Can Do at Home to Awaken the Inner Healer, 2nd edition.

Shadow Hero Workbook, Lessons to purify the Hero archetype in you; Healthy vs. Unhealthy Hero behavior; Unconscious Patterns 201

Adequate and Sufficient Psychic Self-protection; For Healers and Energy Medicine Practitioners

Expanding Human Senses from 5 to 12; Rudolf Steiner's 12 Senses to VAKOG to KAVOG

Muscle Testing for Success; Muscle-testing exercises applied to success topics. Simultaneously published as Success Kinesiology, Dowsing for Success and Muscle Testing for Success. All editions virtually the same except for unique covers.

Unconscious Patterns 101, Tools for the Hero's Journey of Self-healing. Picking up where NLP metaprograms left off, expanding the topic in the context of 'God is my Partner.'

Breast Cancer & Over-giving; Therapeutic Metaphors for Women's Issues (99 cent long article)

Your Habit Body, An Owner's Manual Our habits are our best friends; why then, do we make the same errors over and over again?

"**Willingness to heal** is the pre-requisite for all healing" revised edition coming 2014

The Inner Court: Close-up of the Habit Body

Radical Cell Wellness—Especially for women! Cell psychology for everyone; A coherent theory of illness and wellness

The Five Puberties, Growing new eyes to see children afresh

You have FIVE bodies PACME; Spiritual Geography 101 (99 cent booklet)

The Meaning of Illness is Now an Open Book, Cross-referencing illness and issues

Welcome!

Our meridians are one of several, natural 'Inner Dashboards' available to manage and tweak our sub- and unconscious Your meridians can indeed become your Healing Toolbox.

Find here the best guesses to date of therapeutic metaphors relevant to our 12 meridians and two vessels. Disturbances are further organized by undercharge~overcharge, over-energy and under-energy in Neuroenergetic Kinesiology (NK) terms.

If you know a meridian is disturbed, not flowing in forward direction, stuck or confused, now you can find language to better comprehend how it's disturbed, in accessible mental-emotional terms.

From the other end, if you perceive how a patron is dysfunctional in their feeling and thinking, you can learn which meridian-organ(s) are likely disturbed.

The healthy, balanced expression of each meridian in the human psyche is listed in each section and collated into a list in **To Learn More**.

This is a technique-agnostic manual for traveling back and forth between meridian-organ dysfunction and mental-emotional dysfunction. It's useful for anyone who believes disturbances in our higher frequency bodies trickle down and precipitate into health concerns in our lower frequency physical body.

This manual condenses and improves on the categories and insights of William F. Whisenant's 400 page, *Psychological Kinesiology* (1994). Added to it are many observations from the private practices of the author and other practitioners and sources. Your comments and additions are invited.

Q: Why aren't these Tools That Heal better known?

A: In the field of personal growth and transformation, these are "power tools." Not appropriate to use them outside an ecumenical spiritual framework of 'God is my Partner.' Not appropriate to use them outside of the Law of Spiderman, "With great power goes great responsibility." Not appropriate to use them outside the Law of Gentleness for Healers.

About 100 years from now, more persons; probably coming out of diverse churches and spiritual groups, will have adequate-sufficient foundations in morals, ethics and truly human values, to use and share these Tools safely.

A word about shame, self-doubt, guilt, regret

These cancel healthy self-esteem. Shame and healthy self-esteem cannot co-exist; they are matter and anti-matter; one cancels the other.

Shame is corrupted self-esteem, self-esteem turned against its owner. Shame disturbs our Conception Vessel, our Sea of Yin, on the front of our body.

Shame is contraction where natural healthy self-esteem is personal expansion. Inner Sunshine is a useful metaphor for healthy self-esteem.

The 1980s taught us to increase our self-esteem by repeating affirmations.

Affirmations are additive, thru repetition they add programming and conditioning to our sub- and unconscious; in a word, "entrainment."

This is the weak way to increase healthy self-esteem. The stronger way to do it is with a subtractive processes. Reducing shameful memories automatically expands our natural psychic space for healthy self-esteem.

Why? Healthy self-esteem is the natural state before we became disturbed by things we allowed, promoted or created. Health is always the biggest Pattern. Each cell our immune system creates knows what health is and how to keep contributing to health.

John-Roger says, "It takes great courage to see the face of God. why? Because first you have to see your own face." This points to the courage needed to face-up to where our sub- and unconscious are disturbed and can be redeemed. What's your willingness to heal? Individuals demonstrate their willingness to heal by the the time and attention they invest in using methods of self-connection and self-healing.

Using this manual

Q: Why does the average person feel ill-equipped to discern and address their our own mental-emotional disturbances?

A: Academic and Big Pharma psychology is stuck in an 1800s male paradigm of "psychology as a set of diseases and disorders." Holistic-humanistic psychology which became more mainstream after 1970, was a huge improvement.

I don't expect holistic-humanistic psychology to become more mainstream unless-until wise women occupy more leadership positions in these fields Even holistic-humanistic psychology 1965-1995 was more mired in "neck-up only" abstractions, dis-interested in self-connection; and, how every energy frequency in our waking psyche has its unique intelligence and function to contribute.

Holistic healthcare, practiced in chiropractic, holistic TCM and Energy Medicine, were the first healthcare methods in modern times demonstrating more willingness to connect with the lower two-thirds of our psyche, our sub- and unconscious, the lower two-thirds of our waking psyche:

Waking	- Talking	Creative intellect & analysis
Dreaming	- Feeling	Creative connecting intelligence
Sleeping	- Needing	Creative self-care, self-healing

dg-talk-feel-need

Messages from the Body by Michael Lincoln

For those wishing to connect the dots between illness and mental-emotional issues, *Messages from the Body* by Michael Lincoln, is recommended as a practical desk reference. Terms familiar to counselors, therapists and practitioners are always appreciated.

The better you are at self-muscle-testing, or self-testing of any kind, the more useful *Messages* and the present manual become. Readers can simply test thru the observations-options on a single disturbance, until you find which observation(s) applies most to you now, or to your client.

Physical symptomology is specifically avoided in this text. Physical symptoms mentioned in *Whisenant*, the main source text, have largely been deleted. Matthew Thie's Muscle Metaphors are added for reference from *Touch for Health 2nd Ed.*

This manual arose out of my practice as a Health Intuitive. Anyone in my field frequently puts on a Sherlock Holmes deerstalker hat and wants to know, "Precisely what kind of negativity is present?"

Clear BOTH under- and over-charge

Many disturbed organs and meridians have BOTH under- and overcharge disturbances. I suggest you clear BOTH over- and undercharge and in this order.

OVERcharge is usually compensating for UNDERcharge. If you fill in the "hole" of the under, the over will calm down in time automatically. Use testing to ascertain any further detail desired.

Questions to ask your meridians

One of the reasons a complete meridian psychology had to wait till the 1990s or later was muscle testing had yet to be much applied to meridian disturbances. Since the 1990s we know better questions to ask:

- Is this meridian disturbed? Is this meridian in balance, yes or no?)

- Is the RIGHT (left) bilateral meridian disturbed?

- Is the meridian disturbed *bilaterally* or not? If the meridian IS disturbed *bi*laterally this always suggests the associated organ is disturbed; or possibly, is the cause of the disturbed meridians

- Is the meridian flowing in the healthy direction of flow? (yes or no)

- Is the meridian OVERcharged (UNDERcharged)? Is it both?

- Is it also running backwards? Is it stuck and not moving?

- Is the meridian **element** disturbed? Is it beneficial to check the other meridians of the same element now?

Maybe you can add questions to this list.

Once you uncover conditions relevant to your circumstance, the 'discovery-uncovery' phase is complete. then it's time for solutions. Use what you have in your own Healing Toolbox; use any method on the Energy Medicine Skill Ladder you enjoy experimenting with.

Note ~ While I honor Bradley Nelson of *Emotion Code* for uncovering magnets as an effective method for clearing energetic disturbance, I prefer and recommend self-forgiveness as a safer, more effective method of clearing meridian disturbance.

Slow-Motion Self-Forgiveness is a method of forgiving I use with virtually every client and on myself. It's effective because all our "issues" are habits; all we have is "habits;" 95% of what is present in our sub- and unconscious. All habits are formed thru repetition. Forgive all the repetitions, you clear the habit. This is the value of subtracting in healing. Forgiving is the easiest form of subtraction in self-healing. After subtracting, after releasing, we add or create a new pattern, a new habit. See *Slow-Motion Forgiveness* in its own booklet.

See also "Using the Light to balance meridians and vessels;" and, Two Case Studies in **To Learn More**.

More tools if desired

Mimi Castellanos can be reached http://www.BravoCoop.com

An audio file for clearing the meridians using the Light of the Whole Spirit is easy to make.

William F. Whisenant's *Psychological Kinesiology*

This manual condenses William F. Whisenant's *Psychological Kinesiology* (1994), Monarch Butterfly Productions, Kailua, Hawaii. This seminal work was the first and so far only work I can find to move TCM meridian psychology forward from where it was stuck. TCM had accurate yet extremely limited and elementary language for emotions absorbed by organs. Since the 1990s, the potential was bigger.

Meridians as a thumbnail of our psyche in illness & wellness

Back 100 years at least, the seven "chakras" (wheels) dominated the history of energy anatomy. Now, "etheric centers" is the more polite term replacing "charkas."

Prior to *Whisenant*, 1994, the language of meridians was mostly a bunch of esoteric indications translated from Hindu and Chinese texts. Our chakras are much DEEPER in our unconscious than our meridians and two main vessels. Our chakras are deeper by design. Why? So we don't muck round with them and mess things up in our ignorance.

Our meridians and vessels are much HIGHER in our psyche, in our SUBconscious, closer to the surface of our psyche than our chakras. This is by design. Our meridians are a dashboard humans have opportunity and privilege to work with and master, if they choose to. This is by design.

Our meridians and two main vessels can also be likened to an "operating system," "control panel" for our psyche and unconscious. Meridians are one place to check when a disturbance or health concern does not respond to what you know or to book-learning. The breakthrough language was *Whisenant*, 1994.

Not until *Whisenant* did we get the whole picture, the whole package, of how each vessel-meridian is a reference point, a landmark in the 3D hologram of our psyche. Whisenant went further to uncover or suggest accurate mythological correspondences bridging the meridians-vessels into archetypes many counselors and therapists already had some use for.

My own story? Prior to Whisenant's book, I had been stumbling around in a daze for ten years mumbling, "Where is the correspondence between 20th century humanistic psychology and acupuncture vessels-meridians?"

John Diamond had made the connection between these two, yet, only as a principle, in the abstract. Whisenant's book was not only the first book detailing mental-emotional meanings of meridians, it's the most thoro. NK may be more comprehensive now. At 400 pages of text and photos, *Psychological Kinesiology* is likely his PhD thesis. It's masterful, a wide highway of clarity. It is organized around the meridians, with other material. It has photos of models, case studies, therapeutic metaphors and correspondences in cell salts, exercise, etc. *Whisenant* shows thoro scholarship, commenting on all the more partial works in the field, as of 1994.

Whisenant's good work on sorting psychological phenomena into over- and undercharge categories of expression has been extended and completed here. Additions are added from ten years of personal and clinical work by the author; and, insights of other practitioners who could add to Whisenant's original directness and clarity. Producing this book has been educational for me.

One of many surprises here is we had much more and precise language for psychic pathology than we thought. The key was to organize pathology by under and over-charge.

Comments, corrections, additions, deletions all welcome. Email me.

Where is Whisenant now?

Whisenant is no longer reachable at his Hawaii address or phone. His clinic's phone belongs to someone else. I believe he is in the U.S. I found an email for him and invited him to contribute to this effort--but no response so far. All I can say is "Thanks, Bill! Call me if I can ever assist you!"

Since Whisenant is unavailable for sessions or training, I suggest interested individuals contact practitioners in the following professional-grade modalities, in no particular order:

- Touch for Health (T4H),

- Neuroenergetic Kinesiology (NK),

- Donna Eden's meridian tracing,

- Peace Theological Seminary MSS-DSS,

-Bradley Nelson's Emotion Code,

- BodyTalk

If you get stuck, give me a call.

The energy moving thru all meridians

Etheric energy. Between our imaginal (astral) and physical body, we have Rudolf Steiner's "etheric formative forces." Slowed down towards the frequency of physical tissues, etheric energy differentiates and takes on the qualities of the classical elements. These then appear in our energetic makeup in our meridians.

Is etheric energy the same as nerve energy? Is all nerve energy really etheric energy? In about 100 years this is probably how it will be taught: nerve energy is electricity-*like*. Nerve energy has many of the same characteristics as electricity. Despite Rudolf Steiner and Ernst Lehrs, the ethical, moral, values development simply isn't here yet for etheric topics to become more mainstream. Another hundred years is what John-Roger estimated.

Whisenant does not take on the task of updating five element concepts to five qualities, etc. NK seems to have done the most of this building out of more modern conceptions of what TCM gave us to start with.

WHY do Living cells absorb unresolved hurts?

Hurts, disappointments, perceived betrayals, rejections, and abandonments--all come at us wherever souls take on physical bodies.

Our child within expects our healthy conscious Chooser Self to process these "slings and arrows of outrageous fortune" as it can get to them. This is easier said than done. Without self-connection it's difficult. Even with self-connection, without tools-methods it's challenging. Everyone reading knows the difficulty of processing dramatic and/or traumatic experiences, in the moment they occur, without resorting to habitual reactions.

We provide ourselves needed time for processing and closure via spiritual exercises, rest, sleep, and Energy Medicine experiments. If we don't take time for this; and say, "I'll get to this one later," our child within saves the unresolved energies, puts them 'on the shelf' for later expected processing.

Significant hurts and upsets we do not process and resolve, do not simply evaporate. They have to go somewhere. The Angels created virtually infinite storage capacity in our unconscious Habit Body for when we are unable; or choose, to not to process our hurts.

Our inner child, our habit body, has the job of storing these 'undigested experiences' until such time as we get around to consciously processing them. In the meantime, our child within, our memory body, has as one of its functions, accepting, absorbing, recording and holding onto unresolved hurts, until the soul takes time out from the outer world to devote to inner processing.

If left unresolved for a long time, undigested mental-emotional disturbances accumulate. These are held in sub- and unconscious depths in our psyche. This is 'our baggage,' the psychic clutter we mean to get around to--but for many people--seldom do.

The price we pay for carrying around undigested, unresolved mental-emotional hurts is, over time, our meridians become disturbed. When both bilateral meridians of an organ are disturbed, the associated organ(s) becomes disturbed.

Let's look at the cell level. When our cells absorb negativity, they have less freedom to access nutrients and life energy. Cells can multi-task—but only at a chemical-molecular level. It challenges cells to be both optimally healthy AND be the librarian of thousands of unresolved mental-emotional hurts and upsets.

Physical pain tells us our cells are breaking down from holding onto more unresolved hurts than they can carry. This is usually when we seek out a practitioner for assistance and relief.

When our sub-conscious gets full, they begin to be pushed down into the UNconscious. Our Habit Body does us the favor of stashing unresolved hurts 'down below.' New incoming unresolved hurts get piled on top. Over time the lowest ones get pushed down lower and deeper in *frequency*. When they get pushed down to the low frequency of our meat and bone body--voila!--we have successfully manifested a disease or chronic condition.

Q: Why do our cells absorb and hold onto negativity?

A: Because they are receptive.

Cells resonate more with our kidney *yin* side of consciousness, the "egg" the "container" side of our psyche, before the egg is broken by the masculine, breaking out and stepping forward.

You, me and you, when we are awake, are on the YANG side of consciousness. We are only on the *yin* side of consciousness while we are meditating with a peaceful mind or asleep. The *yin* side of our psyche is relatively asleep compared to our YANG side This is by design. The polarity is by design. Our job as Waking Conscious Self is to bridge everywhere unhelpful gaps exist between the many opposed internal parts of our waking psyche.

North Americans may be the most out of balance. YANG tends to dominate so completely, our *yin* side becomes a big mystery and no one talks about it. This is why the biggest sport in the USA is not baseball, football or basketball. *It's blaming the other guy* (thanks to Wayne Baird, DC for this). For more on this pattern, see Hugo Tobar on Five Qualities (elements) Emotions.

Q: Is this why yoga is so big in the USA, developing receptive *yin* to balance the endless YANG-banging?

A: Yes, especially for women. If you judge or divorce your preferences from healthy *yin*, it takes longer to heal.

Fortunately more Tools That Heal are being practiced on Earth today than at any prior time in Earth's history. The Skill Ladder of Energy Medicine methods-techniques-arts displays these. Experiments are available for every skill level. Okay to compose your own Skill Ladder.

Check Depth of issue

How can we hold both over- and under-charge in a single meridian? Simple. We are creative on three levels:

- conscious,

- sub-conscious and

- unconscious.

These are not metaphors. This is like one of those tall glass cylinders where liquids of differing densities self-organize in a vertical column.

20th century psychology led people to think about our psyche in only the most abstract, intellectual, language-oriented ways. The lower two-thirds of our waking psyche is not limited to what males like to think about and what they say.

More often, overcharge disturbances are on top (Protectors in Internal Family Systems). These are at a higher frequency level. Classically, they compensate for under-charge held at a lower frequency level. This is the energetics behind TopDog and Underdog in Gestalt.

Conscious issues we process by thinking them thru and talking them out. Talk therapy can work, sometimes best with the local bartender or over the back yard fence with a neighbor--but it's slow.

Subconscious issues require slowing down, getting down on on knee to talk with your three year old self. Problematically counselors, coaches and practitioners can't assist patrons to heal any deeper than the depth of their own self-healing. Then personal change goes faster.

In other words, if you want to go faster in your self-healing--slow down.

More on the pattern of subconscious issues aligning right and left in our body, can be found in *The NEW Energy Anatomy.*

A complete theory of illness is beyond our scope here. Find more discussion in *Radical Cell-Wellness-Especially for Women!*

We need each other to heal. When we encounter new disturbances, previously unknown to us, we need sisters and brothers who have already resolved the hurts we are encountering for the first time.

Organs and meridians connect energetically

For the purposes of self-healing, it helps to imagine organs and their associated meridians as energetically equal. You can treat either one, by means of the other. Simply find the priority direction to work in: Does this client's own Higher Guidance suggest we start with the organs and work towards the meridians? Or, does this client's own Higher Guidance suggest we start with the meridian disturbance and work towards the organs?

More precisely, two levels of frequency connect. Meridians are the organs at a higher frequency. Organs are the meridians at a lower frequency.

This is why energetically the issues of both tend to coincide. A lifetime of experiences with treating people thru meridians--experience I do not have--is called for to verify this. It wasn't my path; maybe it's your path.

No one would confuse cellular tissues of a physical organ with the energetic flow of a meridian. However, grasp the charge and flow in a meridian, and you understand the health or disturbed nature of the associated organ.

Alexander Holub's book, *Psychokinesiology* (Bridger House, 1999) was instrumental in convincing me the emotions absorbed by a meridian overlap virtually 100% with emotions absorbed by corresponding organs. The striking similarity of emotions in an organ-meridian pairs is NOT imaginary!

Bilateral meridian imbalance points to organic organ disturbance

I found this wisdom in my Touch for Health notes. Happy to give more precise credit if I knew the source. Worth adding here is bilateral imbalance does not guarantee organic damage or disturbance; the disturbance can be primarily energetic. The game is to find latent energetic disturbances and clear them before they do manifest physically.

Overview of undercharge & overcharge

Undercharge & overcharge in meridians & organs

Despite a lack of clarity in literature before *Whisenant* (1994), a theory of under and overcharge is a surprisingly easy concept to articulate using water metaphors. At its simplest...

undercharge = empty of any flow

Overcharge = overflowing, too much flow

To make this useful for self-healing, transpose the water metaphors into mental-emotional behaviors-expressions:

Undercharge = feeling empty, alone, low self care, neglected, over-relaxed; hence, related to low blood pressure and emotional neglect.

Overcharge = overflowing, unnecessarily aggressive, wound up, too 'out there,' hyped up, over-reactive; hence, related to high blood pressure and potent unresolved issues boiling just below the surface of awareness.

Meridian overcharge

Poetically, overcharge is too much water for the stream bed, a flood! Overcharge is everything suggested by excess yang, any behavior perceived as "too much," overly forceful behavior of any kind, like overselling.

Overcharge is dramatically on display in old-time hellfire and brimstone preaching and evangelizing. The famous "Type A" personality, the driven go-getter, gotta-gotta, go-go, stress-stress. These are people over-identified with overcharged element-meridian expressions.

True Darth Vader expressions, not parodies, are overcharge. James Cameron's Terminator robots are archetypes of overcharge. Terminator robots get beat up, shot, maimed yet take no interest in their own welfare, no attention given nor expected from their own capacity for self-healing. This is overcharge divorced--and often judgmental of--yin-nourishing, yin-healing forces.

Speaking more generally, overcharge is greed, ambition, and excesses of the seven deadly sins: extravagance, later lust, gluttony, greed, envy, pride.

The only undercharge sin is sloth. The rest of the classic sins are all over-exuberance of the basic self, connected with willfulness and willpower, the basic self is out of balance towards YANG. Why? Over-doing of YANG to compensate for under-nourished *yin*. Classic.

Meridian undercharge

UNDERcharge examples ~ Undercharge is too little water flowing in the stream bed, a drought! Overcharge is everything suggested by *yin* deficiency, lack of "smiling energy," lack of gentle, radiant, Inner Sunshine.

Undercharge is emptiness where there should be substance, a hole in the road needing filling in level with surrounding ground. The energetic of homelessness, empty of life, empty of self-nurturing. Underpowered expressions of all kinds.

Try to keep these two really simple because they are simple. Do not conflate with gender. Over- and undercharge translate *poorly* into male~female.

Simple is: depression is undercharge. Hypertension, feeling driven for no reason, is overcharge. Too little or too much.

The words above point to things you might feel consciously. Meridians and organs also get "depressed" and "hyper" (more precisely, they get habituated one way or the other). This activity occurs SUBconsciously. Practice with these terms on your self and become more aware of these highs and lows "behind the scenes," the ups and downs "swept under the rug."

Clear both over- and undercharge in each session

Whenever a meridian is disturbed, more often than not it has both over and undercharge imbalances. Looking for both is wise. Overcharges clear faster and easier when you clear undercharge first. This seems to be the natural sequence: The under has to come up before the over can calm down. Over- was high to to begin with to compensate for under- being low.

Overcharged meridians can't calm down because they compensate for deficiencies in undercharged meridians and organs.

This why increasing our own self-care, taking care of our own needs, first, last and always, increasing nourishing *yin*, is such effective therapy. It reduces the need for over-doing of all kinds.

Piano wire metaphor for under-overcharge

A taught piano wire at rest is at peace, neither vibrating to the left nor to the right. Pluck it. Does it vibrate just to the left? Or does it always vibrate bilaterally, to BOTH left and right sides; and, to both sides more or less equally? Same with meridians.

Axis of dysfunction for each meridian

Dysfunctional expressions in meridians, organs and vessels can be discerned to be either undercharged, overcharged; or both.

Axis of dysfunction is a pattern similar to polar opposites: both poles are dysfunctional, neither are functional nor desirable. The goal is neither black nor white but workable, agreeable middle ground between both extremes.

In conventional terms we say 'healthy homeostasis is in the middle.' Rudolf Steiner might say, the healthy, alive, feelingful position is often found in the middle ground between two positions.

"There is no black and white. There is only color" ~ Douglas Rushkoff

Three illustrative examples:

Governing Vessel (self-concept meridian) ~ Over-concentrated focus and intensity, over-doing life; at the other end, "Whatever. I'll do it tomorrow," never any urgency ever at all. Unhealthy complacency. The middle ground is clearly healthy engagement, not too intense; nor, too detached, too limp, too uninvolved.

Pericardium Meridian (generosity & gratitude meridian, previously: "Circulation-Sex") ~ Numbing out on passive addictions. At the other end, flying off the handle in reckless over-activity. The middle ground is clearly healthy engagement and rhythmic reciprocity, both doing for others; and, arranging to get your own needs met.

Triple Warmer Meridian (also: Triple Warner)~ Heaviness, depression; at the other end, exaggerated lightness, ungrounded, unacknowledged mania. The middle ground is clearly mindful caution and estimation of where taking healthy risks verges into danger.

The healthy balance (homeostasis) of a meridian or organ will always be somewhere in this range between two unhealthy extremes; hence, the idea of an axis of dysfunction.

-=+ -=+ -=+ -=+ -=+ -=+ -=+ -=+ -=+

A few words on Governing & Conception Vessels

Headline: The energetic spine for the inner child is in front. Physically it includes our esophagus and tongue. As a child, our sense of well-being and self-esteem are very tied to our front "spine." Our front spine follows our Conception Vessel.

The energetic spine for the conscious Self is in back. In our awake psyche this is our self-concept. Our back spine follows our Governing Vessel.

Our 12 meridians lie primarily in our SUBconscious. Our two Vessels are deeper in our UNconscious.

If energy activity in our meridians and vessels was consciously perceptible by the average person, perceptions of where energy is flowing or blocked could become very distracting as hundreds of changes occur every day.

If you personally are already awake to some of the energy changes inside you, on a daily basis, most of what you are perceiving is likely meridian activity in your SUB- and UNconscious.

Our two vessels are characterized poetically in TCM as, "GV is the sea of yang; CV is the sea of yin."

It appears GV and CV do not have as strong direction of flow as each of the 12 meridians do. The GV in back is especially problematic to interfere with in any way. Our GV vessel, like our DNA, is by design "out of reach" of the conscious self so we don't muck around and screw things up.

The two vessels on the front and back of our body can be likened to two vertical columns of Light in the body. A "two-way street" permits energy to move either up or down compared to a "one way street."

In some TCM charts these two vessels have dedicated directions of flow. More useful to me seems to be de-emphasizing direction of flow for these two meridians. Direction of flow appears to be subservient to the capacity of these vessels to "stand" for their respective energy, magnetic in front, electric in back. This does not contradict the poetry of "sea of yin" and "sea of yang." We experience our electric and magnetic potentials dimly, as if in a dream, if at all.

The two vessels are less conditioned than the meridians; they are more archetypal, closer to our unconscious and its attention to needs. The deeper levels of our habit body contain habits set in motion "at the factory," by angels, if you will.

They say, "You can't change the spots on a leopard." Fortunately this is only true of leopards. Humans can change their spots—but you have to really want to, high willingness to heal and to change for the better makes this possible--then, persistence and perseverance. If you have courage to change your own "spots," your own supposedly indelible markings--where do you find them? You find them here in the sub- and unconscious.

CV-GV as front and back of the body

Leaving aside our skeleton for the moment, the front of our body is characterized by the Conception Vessel.

The back of our body is characterized by the Governing Vessel.

GV resonates with our capacity for healthy concentrated attention, alertness and with-it-ness. GV resonates with the cerebral nervous system (brain, spine, lateral spinal nerves).

CV resonates with our capacity for healthy relaxation in our vagus nerve, front and back.

Hence our body has significant potential difference, front & back. A dynamic balance is the goal. If you think of GV and CV each as one hand, the goal is to able to use "both hands" alternately as useful.

Overcharge in the GV looks like an unnecessarily rigid body, rigid role playing, rigid emotions, rigid beliefs—a "dam" holding back low self-esteem in the personal life. Batman Dark Knight among other images.

A common chiropractic diagnosis fits here. When abdominal muscles *in front* are weak from lack of exercise, the low back muscles *in back* tighten up. Same pattern.

Contrast in charge between our front and back is healthy, up to a point. A key to moderating overcharge in GV is to address and support undercharged disturbances. Why? Overcharge is compensating for weak undercharge.

See more on this in *The NEW Energy Anatomy; Nine new views of the human psyche. No clairvoyance required.*

See 'Clark Kent and Superman in action' below as the major myth of paired dysfunction on front and back of the body.

CV as your self-esteem vessel

We experience our front vessel as self-esteem.

A more modern name for the Conception Vessel is the Self-esteem vessel. Our "Sea of Self-esteem" develops in utero to just before puberty.

GV as your self-concept vessel

We experience our back vessel as self-esteem.

A more modern name for the Governing Vessel is the Self-concept vessel. Our healthy self-concept develops emerges or develops after puberty.

CV and GV together as self-confidence

Front of body = Conception Vessel = self-esteem

Back of body = Governing Vessel = self-concept

> Healthy self-esteem + healthy self-concept = healthy self-confidence

Self-esteem and self-concept together add up to self-confidence. This is a precise and useful characterization of these vessels.

Notice this works backwards too:

Low self-confidence in the Conception Vessel, in the front of the body, expresses as low self-esteem.

Low self-confidence expresses in the Governing Vessel, in the back of the body, expresses as low self-concept.

Our human pattern is self-esteem, in front, suffers and becomes deficient (undercharge). Then self-concept, in back, becomes exaggerated (overcharge) to compensate.

These two vessels are perhaps always dysfunctional as a pair; leading to the insight: self-esteem and self-concept are often out of whack as a pair. More on this further below.

Dysfunction in the CV looks like hiding and scatter in the unconscious

Dysfunction in the GV looks like unnecessary rigid muscles, rigid role playing (Batman again), rigid emotions and rigid beliefs in the unconscious.

CV-GV together are crucial dimensions of how good I feel about myself, how Coherent, Integrated and Aligned (CIA) I am when awake in my body.

Dysfunction in the GV looks like dissociation, excess pride and arrogance

An overly positive self-image can be over-charge in the Governing Vessel. Batman feels his overcharge as "strength." Batman mis-perceives and mis-understands.

Excess charge in GV can be de-escalated, calmed down, by activating healthy vagal nerve tone. The way this looks socially is listening to others, listening to feedback on how we come across; and ultimately, by exercising compassion, caring and empathy.

CV as magnetic, GV as electric

Someone online remarked "the CV is magnetic in nature and the GV is electric in nature." After living with this for some time, growing "new eyes" to see if this is true or not, I find this is indeed a window on a true phenomena.

We consciously perceive strong human magnetism in visual media of seductive females. Seduction is one "talent" of magnetism on the front of our body. You can find striking imagery of women's magnetic consciously mobilized in any video commercial for Victoria Secret underwear. Notice all the "come hither" tropes. This "certain something," this "sex appeal" is a hallmark of magnetic energy. It draws you in—magnetic. The singer Madonna used to embody very magnetic CV energy.

The tropes of the woman walking straight at the viewer, looking straight at the viewer, this is GV electricity.

Magnetic energy is not bad. It's just energy. The purposes you harness it too determine it's value. Healthy magnetism can be used for intimacy, closeness, nurturing and especially to support children and those in need of support. It's also half of our physical regeneration ability. Apart from sex, keeping our CV healthy is part of our self-care.

The other half is our electric capacity. This is harder to see and harder to see in cultures where healthy male energy harnessed to ethical projects, goals, and issues is in short supply. Habitat for Humanity is a good exception. Attend any HH housebuilding and you will find lots of men, working cooperatively, swatting nails into boards and running wires to and from electrical boxes. They behave with purpose, energy and determination. They are having fun and they are fun to be with. In construction work, males often demonstrate GV electrical potential used for positive purposes.

Another place to find healthy GV expressions is to go back to Thomas Paine, the Declaration of Independence and Howard Zinn's *Voices of a People's History of the United States: Second Edition*, especially the audio versions. You will hear the intensity, focus and determination of intention focused on goals beneficial to the 99%.

This topic suggests the possibility all yang meridians are electric in nature and all *yin* meridians magnetic in nature. This seems likely to be true.

CV as gut brain, GV as head brain

CV resonates with our gut brain, which is below and in front in our body.

GV resonates with our cerebral brain, which is above and behind in our body.

The enteric nervous system (ENS), the gut brain, is in the lower torso, below the diaphragm muscle. This is the main physiology of the habit body, inner child, immune system, feeling mind, and *dan tien*.

The cerebral nervous system (CNS), is nerve tissue in the brain, spine and nerves radiating from the spine, virtually all above our dome-shaped diaphragm muscle. This is the physiology of the conscious self, rational mind, waking cognition, the "light of day" in our psyche.

Consider this *over*-simplification: our gut brain resonates more with Feelings. Our head brain resonates more with Thinking.

Consider this simplification. What if this is as simple as our waking experience matching a thought with a feeling; and alternately, matching feelings with thoughts. John-Roger has pointed to this as a major expression of an integrated psyche.

CV and GV somehow connect and integrate unconscious aspects of our two brains in deeper ways than the 12 elemented meridians. Exactly how, is somewhat unique to each individual so hard to generalize about and not so useful to generalize about. Best way to explore this and learn about it is case by case, client by client.

Q: What about the Man Tak Chia topic, the "microcosmic orbit."

A: Neither myself nor my healing buddy are in favor of this practice. We have found it more problematic for Westerners than helpful. Much more useful and practical is working on practicing interpersonal competency and connecting with your vagus nerve if you are an over-achiever of any kind.

CV-GV are crucial dimensions of how good I feel about myself, top and bottom in my body.

-=+ -=+ -=+ -=+ -=+ -=+ -=+ -=+ -=+

CONCEPTION VESSEL

(Also called Central Meridian)

No element YIN

Muscles from Touch for Health: Supraspinatus

Healthy, positive, balanced: It's easy and natural for me to be, do and express creatively here in the 3D world.

Other healthy expressions: Sensitivity to opportunity in front of me, in both time and space, to create, express and conceive new creations, sensing personal opportunity to give birth to new things here in 3D.

Negative emotions absorbed: low self-esteem. Perceived inability to create and manifest in the 3D world and/or in relationships. "If you knew what I was really like, you wouldn't want me." Therefore, hiding and hiding out, afraid to come out of the closet and be yourself. Scatter, too many irons in the fire, nothing getting completed or resolved. Spaced-out, New Age Space Case. This really does seem to be scattering of the CV energies so they cannot ground here in 3D.

UNDER- pole dysfunction: All deficits of self-esteem (not to be confused with deficits of self-concept), shame, given up, scattered, inwardly disconnected, confused, shy, in overwhelm, emotionally neutered. An unending "culture of personal crisis" as reported by Max Blumenthal in Republican Gomorrah (2009).

UNDER- myths: Fails to cultivate romantic aspects of relationships. Fails to make much money, have fun, have children, play with and enjoy children.

The underdog who retreats to an alternative version of reality. Walter Mitty in the "The Secret Life of Walter Mitty (1939)," his non-fantastic self.

May not be actively self-destructive but if anger is also present extreme cases have a strong possibility of suicide attempt. Homeless persons destroying themself thru self-neglect. Attention to support system may be so poor they literally waste away.

End of life issues. Abandons all activities in life calling for self-assertion.

OVER- pole dysfunction: Any kind of "faking it," putting on and keeping up appearances, faking-pretending-imagining high self-esteem as in the motif of the masked super hero.

Other OVERcharged expressions: Playing roles, performing rituals and routines to compensate for low self-esteem.

All schizophrenics have dysfunctional CV, a disintegrated sense of self (*Whisenant*).

Myth for the CV ~ Clark Kent as 98 pound weakling. This myth is covered in the CV GV myth section below.

If we had Conception Vessel at all

Infinite, constant unworthiness. Never feel worthwhile, so not very capable of action.

If we had no Governing Vessel at all

We would be completely controllable by someone else's self-image, like a zombie disciple of a guru, who can do no more nor less than what the Master tells them. No values, no personal preferences of your own, only the Master's values. Not pleasant.

Other energetic CV lore

+ Zip Up: Because our CV is magnetic, it easily becomes congested, polluted, disturbed, too-open or too-exposed to the influence of other beings. Zip Up invites you to close your psychic field in a healthy way, to re-establish your healthy magnetic boundaries. You always zip UP on CV-GV vessels, I suggest in front, zip up to the lower lip. Do this three times. This technique is useful before speaking in front of crowds or to a person you know is angry. Donna Eden demonstrates this on many Youtube videos.

+ Undercharged CV is closely related to the underdog position in the poles of topdog-underdog in Gestalt Therapy.

Pattern of Conception Vessel dysfunction: giving up my power to an external something, some sacred cow, giving my inner authority/center over to:

physical pleasure, sexual pleasure

an addiction

a compulsion

a quest for power (over others)

a quest for human loves

an undefined search

material success, material wealth

Possible issues with self, family & friends, other people, world and how you connect with your own Divinity.

+ The central meridian is where the used energy of the other meridians is stored prior to being released with the breath on exhaling (Matthew Thie).

+ Dominates the *yin* of the whole body; therefore, described as the Sea of Yin Meridians. This is poetic way of saying the above: CV is the most unconscious of all *yin* meridians. The three *yin* meridians of the hand and the three *yin* meridians of the foot all join at CV 3. This meridian originates in the uterus and is especially connected with conception.

Its function is regulating circulation of blood and Qi in the *yin* meridians. Regulates the menstrual flow. Dominates the reproductive system and the fetus. Regulates the Qi circulation of the chest, promotes the function of spleen and stomach and generally strengthens the body - taiji-qigong.co.uk/Articles/8extra.html

+ If the CV is weak in an individual, look for cords and "puppeteers," stronger personalities who wish to direct and control the client (Mimi). Hence fear is the first tool for dictators, demagogues, anyone wishing to accumulate public psychic energy because fear is toxic to CV and forces people to dissociate from their own life; then, look for a more fulfilling life outside their own self. These will be unconscious connections.

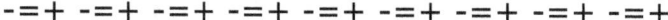

-=+ -=+ -=+ -=+ -=+ -=+ -=+ -=+ -=+

GOVERNING VESSEL

No element YANG

Muscles from Touch for Health: Teres Major

Healthy, positive, balanced: The weather vane. The gauge of environment in adults (CV is gauge of environment before puberty). Will power. Endorphin reactions to various substances. Hearing of intuitive essence in adults. When GV is parallel to and resonating with your own internal, vertical column of Light; then, strong will power, regulated energy, positive inner guidance.

Self-confidence, self-assured stance in life, connected with own personal power without any need to flaunt it, exploit it or boast about it, comfortable standing tall in your own column of Light. Dress up play as children do; playing roles in the sense of relaxed experimentation with new roles and rehearsal, not commitment to any single role—unless it's CIA with your goals, passions and dreams and the highest good for the greatest number.

Easiest polarity to "see" the axis of dysfunction: Over-concentrated focus and intensity, over-doing life; versus, "Whatever." "I'll do it tomorrow," never any urgency or purposefulness at all.

Negative expression - Lack of willingness; stubbornness (over-charged). Overbearing; fluctuating energy; deafness to what is heard inwardly and/or outwardly.

Emotions absorbed: embarrassment, (un)supported, distrust of others, (un)burdened, (dis)integrity.

UNDER- pole dysfunction: fragile sense of own power and self worth

OVER- pole dysfunction: overconfident, inflated sense of own power and worth

Other UNDERcharged behavior: inferiority, distrust self, unrealistic sense of powerlessness, guilt-based self-rejection.

Other OVERcharged behavior: over-confident, throws their weight around.

Myth for both CV and GV

+ In MBTI the classic American psyche of today, was formed between about 1890 and 1960 and is strongly ESTJ. The Horatio Alger stories, of rags to riches, whose author died 1899, are the first expressions of undercharged CV compensated by an over-muscular riches phase expressive of the overcharged GV. Rags = undercharged CV; excessive riches = overcharged GV.

More familiar to readers is the polarity of is a 98 pound weakling Clark Kent; and, the musclebound Superman in action. Debuting in 1939 this polar pair is closely related to the "Secret Life of Walter Mitty," which began as a short story in 1941.

The basic pattern is deficient CV, "98 pound weakling," a reference to famous Charles Atlas muscle building comic book ad where a skinny undercharged boy weakling gets sand kicked in his face by a bully. Clark Kent is this same undercharged weakling image. In this polarity Clark Kent is in front, representing undercharged CV and overcharged GV in back, fantasies of Superman in action.

The 1940s Superman portrays this polarity most clearly. Clark is always in the under-dog position at least somewhat. He constantly misses opportunities to woo and win Lois Lane, get the lead headline, get the glory, etc. He can only win in his alter ego (fantasy).

The gap between how Clark Kent feels about his personal life and how Superman feels saving falling airplanes, measures the distance between overcharge in back (GV) and undercharge in front of the body (CV).

GV overcharge says, "I have to do everything myself, no one else can do what I can, therefore I must act; I am responsible, I had to act!"

Readers who know modern history will know how closely this reflects the United States on the eve of entering WW II. The earlier Great Depression was the U.S. in Clark Kent (low self-esteem) mode. The U.S. leading the Allies and saving Europe is Superman (high self-concept) mode.

Later versions of Clark Kent from the 1950s on show him as stronger and more competent. The contrast between Clark and his alter ego was reduced. Speaking as a myth-maker, if you make both Clark and Supe competent and capable, the character has no subtext at all and becomes bland or a caricature.

Lois Lane in her role as helpless damsel in distress also represents the undercharged CV. Lois in her capable star reporter role is perhaps an echo of Clark's superior alter ego. Rescuing poor helpless bystanders is big business for superheroes, rescuing the poor, undercharged CV.

Superman and Kryptonite ~ Green Kryptonite comes from Kal-El's planet (family) of origin. Green Kryptonite forcefully reminds Superman of his original birth and non-super state by making him weak and removing his super powers. When Green Kryptonite is near, Superman returns to his infantile helpless state, vulnerable and weak again.

This is wonderfully artistic reflection of being suddenly stripped of all GV self-concept enhancers and being reduced to your own true low self-esteem. Life can do this to us: divorce, job loss, death...

Superman comic book scripters have attempted stories where WITHOUT superhuman powers, Superman acknowledging, embracing, unburdening and lifting up his low self-esteem internal parts. To do it justice, this fruitful storyline requires insight and usually the authors personal experience of self-transformation.

The 1940s Superman concept remains the most mythologically interesting for these reasons. See also in this book, discussion of Superman and most superheroes as over~undercharged Triple Warmer Meridian.

Many of the other heroes primarily express only the one side, overcharged GV, the more common North American dysfunction:

- Lone Ranger is primarily overcharged GV. This is why he's so rigid.

- Dick Tracy is tough, rigid, no softness at all.

Batman as a Dark Knight has no Robin to suggest any softness.

These are GV fantasies of pumped-up self concept without any subtext or backstory of the other polarity, the equally dysfunctional, undercharged personal life.

Faith-based self-image ~ This is an extreme version of the Lil' Abner joke, "If it's good for General Bullmose, it's good for the US of A." Faith-based self-image is visible as a lack of flexibility, narrow-mindedness, in the posturing of many regressive social parties, causes and personalities.

Steven Spielberg's Indiana Jones at core remains a kinder, gentler version of Dick Tracy and Lone Ranger. Indiana still works primarily alone, takes all responsibility to himself, has virtually no emotional life, always preferring to run off to catch the next new (imagined) adventure.

Why five year olds like to play dress up and/or wear a cape. This is the same pattern of "I can be somebody!" in a simpler form than the superhero.

Why superheroes have only one power

A big issue for undercharged CV is scatter. A superhero is a more focused self-concept. This is why superheroes commonly only have one power: focus. As a child self-esteem is most easily built by doing one thing well. If one persists, the thrill of mastering one ability, leads to 10,00 hours and to significant mastery.

Why most superheroes wear a mask

A mask means it does not feel safe to be myself, to show my undercharged CV issues. It does not feel safe to FEEL how they feel, to allow others to see "thru the mask" and expose the (undercharge) of the inner child.

The few heroes who do not wear masks, are deeply conflicted about it. Superheroes are about escaping from our undercharged personal lives. When Superman goes into action, our inner Clark Kent is set aside, we turn away from him, Clark disappears when Superman goes into action.

Superhero costumes represent this disappearing act; and also, the more bright, shiny and distinctive persona of the overcharged alter ego. The bright costumes are self-concept on steroids.

The animal rescuer

Let's agree helping animals is a good thing for all of us to do. Let's also agree a few people are identified with being animal rescuers to an unusual degree. What if this is the same the same Superman-Clark Kent polarity? The undercharged front of the body identifies with the weak, helpless, animal. The back of the body identifies itself as the rescuer, who has unusual powers to redeem the animal from its oil-slick, its homelessness, its slaughterhouse, and so on.

Since the 1970s, this pattern of undercharged CV and overcharged GV has evolved somewhat. Interested readers can explore some of the nuances in Lenore Bentz's, *Personality Type, An Owner's Manual* . In the section on the X-Files, she uncovers how the classic U.S. psyche drifted from ESTJ to ENTP in recent generations.

Other energetic GV lore

+ Zip Up: Our GV is much more hidden than our CV. It can still be congested, polluted or disturbed by past actions and choices. Zip Up invites you to close your psychic field in a healthy way, to re-establish your healthy boundaries re self-concept. You always zip UP on CV-GV vessels. On GV, all the way up over the head to top lip. Do this three times. This technique is useful before speaking in front of crowds or to a person you know is angry. I believe this began as a Donna Eden idea.

+ Shushumna, GV and energetic strength are related concepts.

The Shushumna is an exclusively energetic structure visible to some clairvoyants. It exists in a frequency higher than the physical body. A column of Light may describe it. It has no physical function. It appears to be closely related to our inner radiance; and therefore, our energetic strength.

It runs down the body from the head, in front of the spine and behind the physical heart. Ideally it "roots" itself in the first etheric center whereby it connects the person strongly with the Earth, grounding head energies (our spiritual capacities) all the way down into the Earth.

One of my clairvoyant friends says the GV also has no physical function, only an energetic function, absorbing light. The function of these two appears to overlap, possibly to coincide. Secrets of energetic strength appear to be hidden here.

+ TCM idea of GV as "Sea of Yang Meridian."

GV meridian is often referred to as the sea of yang meridians because the three yang meridians of both foot and hand converge into the Du meridian [?] at GV 14. The functions of the GV meridian are to

- regulate the circulation of blood and Qi in the Yang meridians,

- regulate the functional activities of the brain and the spine marrow,

- regulate the function of the urinary and reproductive systems.

(taiji-qigong.co.uk/Articles/8extra.html)

+ Duality held in the unconscious can manifest as unbalanced CV~GV. Deeply held struggle and identification with struggle in delta-unconscious, can manifest as unbalanced CV & GV.

Duality held in the unconscious can manifest as unbalanced CV~GV. Deeply held struggle and identification with struggle in delta-unconscious, can manifest as unbalanced CV & GV.

One pattern of this is CV is high while GV is very low in comparison. Behind this observed measurement is a deeply (delta) unconscious struggle with duality. The human experience in physical form is rife with duality; get used to it; it's normal and natural. The nature of the soul is Oneness, no duality. We are both.

We express all sorts of duality here in the physical and we express oneness as soul. If this is not "okay" with you, there will be an internal struggle; If this paradox is a problem for you, it can show up in these two vessels.

Both CV and GV wish to be strong, like two beautiful, flowering stalks of the same plant. But if an unconscious habit keeps judging duality as bad-wrong-weak, they cannot both be strong. Intolerance of duality here, in any sense channel, KVAOG, will disturb the natural healthy balance of CV~GV.

Mimi C. suggests when the GV comes over the top of the head, towards the top lip, it can go around the nose. If it curves around the nose to the right, it can express as nosyness. This can be a bent towards research, towards bookish study or towards gossip

-=+ -=+ -=+ -=+ -=+ -=+ -=+ -=+ -=+

A few words on the fire element

Lonny Jarrett in *Nourishing Destiny* clarifies the themes of the metaphor of fire. Fire is warmth, expansion; and, also "moving away" from physical materiality. One of our tasks in the physical-material human experience is to identify sufficiently with our survival ego, body deva. It's useful for navigating thru the 3D world. Yet our lower self is not our eternal-immortal soul, not our healthy Self. When fire is over-charged, this can lead to attempts to control, allowing too much emotion, so things and situations devolve into chaos (fire has potential to return matter to energy (chaos).

The dilemma of fire is, on one hand, control is a useful tool, a fire strategy. The individual says, "My desires make me happy." Yet living this way keeps our immortal-eternal soul within Creation. To earn the freedom to be less restricted by Creation, requires practiced self-discipline surrendering desires for more sustainable inner contentment.

People with a strong fire emphasis have the task of transforming attachment to their desires, the wants of the temporary body deva. With practice we learn to surrender compulsive desires and acknowledge the truth of Self leadership, as in Internal Family Systems. As the body deva learns to trust healthy Self-leadership, the anxious over-doing of the body deva calms down.

The under-charge fire challenge is. as we expand and move out and away from materiality, not to go cold and over-detached, to maintain healthy inner warmth (empathy, compassion, etc). As we expand larger and larger, watch inner coldness doesn't take over. Stay with feelings of warm inner contentment.

-=+ -=+ -=+ -=+ -=+ -=+ -=+ -=+ -=+

Pericardium Meridian

Other names: Circulation-sex Meridian, Heart Protector Meridian

Fire Yin

Muscles from Touch for Health:

Gluteus Medius ~ Adductors ~ Piriformis ~ Gluteus Maximus

Warning, this meridian has many names and is often confused with the triple warmer, which it is not. The real alternative names are: Circulation-sex Meridian, Heart protector Meridian, and Heart Constrictor Meridian.

Axis of Dysfunction ~ numbing out on passive addictions; on the other hand, flying off the handle in reckless over-activity (see also "A Few Words..." above).

UNDER- pole dysfunction: addicted to numbing out on gloomy, passive addictions to get away from the anxiety of a crisis of identity. Binge-watching TV is the most modern method.

OVER- pole dysfunction: addiction to active, harsh, reckless, emotional drama (hysteria is the old term) to avoid-deny-escape from the anxiety of a crisis of identity.

Numbness. "Anything to reduce awareness" – *Whisenant*

Your generosity and gratitude meridians

Many readers will know original acupuncture literature stems from a view of human energy which was current 5000 years ago. Among teachers I know, only Rudolf Steiner makes clear how humans were constituted significantly different (more primitively organized) 5000 years ago than we are now.

One 5000 year old view very ripe for updating is the Pericardium Meridian, also called the Circulation-Sex meridian. This meridian-organ has perhaps evolved more than most from how it was perceived in Asia, 5000 years ago, especially in the urban-educated West. If readers know of any other literature on rectifying the pericardium meridian, I'd love to learn of it.

Let's look at the organ level. On the physical organ level, it's unimpressive, a simple 'glove around the heart muscle.' However, in the etheric and astral frequency, the pericardium embodies our capacity for a cornucopia of pink bubble hearts, cute bunnies, kitties, babies, flowers and the honeymoon period of romances.

Q: What about the old Chinese description of the Pericardium meridian as the King's Bodyguard, the heart protector?

A: This was its perceived and actual function in 5000 B.C. in China. 'Heart Protector" imagery describes the primary high point or "aim" of this meridian in the human psyche, 5000 years back. Humankind has evolved so the facts have changed.

In modern terms, the feelings associated with pink hearts, cute bunnies, kitties, babies, flowers and the honeymoon period are positive, uplifting feelings, upward spirals for sure. These feelings around the heart muscle support and protect it from becoming too deadened and mechanical in its rhythmic vortexing of the blood. The uplift of hearts, flowers, babies "protects" the heart muscle from becoming too materialistic, too focussed on only downward spirals.

Pericardium as "Hello Kitty!"

As the heart muscle needed less "protection," it freed up the pericardium to evolve. The pericardium function has evolved towards "Hello Kitty!" "Hello Kitty!" was not a safe, viable psychic option in China in 5,000 BC. "Hello Kitty!" originated in Japan and peaked in the early 2000s. A healthy "Hello Kitty!" function is part of a healthy childhood, age-appropriate around age 9.

Our pericardium enfolds, protects, and "nests" the heart muscle. It is the "swaddling cloth" of our heart muscle, beating within the swaddling. How the Pericardium protects the heart muscle has evolved from the earlier militaristic defensive function, the "king's bodyguard" to the hearts, rainbows and unicorns of adolescent romantic imagery, impulse and feeling.

This unconscious emotional evolution happened most recently for the Japanese people since WW II. I think this is why "Hello Kitty!" is a modern Japanese pop phenomena.

What about "heart constrictor"? Our heart organ itself, the mass of muscle, has evolved and stabilized to where it no longer needs a "heart constrictor" function. Look around, we in the West are plenty constricted in our heart feelings.

Circulation-sex meridian and addictive behavior

I'm not an addiction specialist. I'm going to take a guess here, tho, and suggest the connection between this meridian and addictive behavior, so strongly experienced by William Whisenant in *Psychological Kinesiology* (1994), happens as he describes.

If we have unmet needs; and, we find something fulfilling our needs, if we don't work to heal the deeper unmet need, we will get caught up in and stuck in (addicted) to the feeling of temporary satisfaction provided by our drug of choice (sex, drugs, rock 'n roll, violent video games, etc).

The RHYTHM of generosity and gratitude

Music is much better than words to convey ideas of rhythm. We experience the rhythmic alternation of these two somewhat in lovemaking, when lovers alternate pleasing each other.

Adults often experience this alternation of generosity and gratitude again in nurturing and caring for young children—when things go smoothly.

The Angelic Plan was for the human experience to alternate between generosity and gratitude, as much as possible. On such rhythms successful partnerships, families and communities can be built.

Music to feel and flush Pericardium meridian

Music exists suggesting the Pericardium meridian going both directions.

In the 1990s, the original phenomena of Smooth Jazz, started by 94.7 The Wave in Los Angeles innovated a genre we might call heartfelt music; much of it, healthy pericardium music, music of generosity and gratitude.

Emblematic of healthy pericardium music are The Rippingtons. One piece, "Snowbound" on the album, Curves Ahead, expresses both the healthy downward flow of the meridian; and, then in an interlude about 2/3 thru, the constricted upward flow. The music then returns to healthy downward and outward flow of generosity and gratitude. You may wish to see if you can feel this difference going from healthy to uptight and back to healthy in your meridians.

In effect this one song traces the Pericardium meridians in their healthy direction of flow--reverses, traces them in the opposite direction--then reverse and traces them again in the healthy direction of flow. In Donna Eden's Meridian Tracing, this is called "flushing the meridian."

Your generosity meridian is your RIGHT Pericardium Meridian. When it's flowing down from head towards hand, it's easy to share our heart feelings and give from our overflow.

Giving from obligation is not this, neither is over-giving from a sense of obligation.

Your gratitude meridian is your left Pericardium Meridian. When it's flowing down from head to hand, it's easy to perceive, receive and reach out to get our own needs met.

Feeling deprived, feeling un-met needs, causes the left Gratitude Meridian to flow backwards, "uphill," from hand to head, giving us an "uptight feeling."

The whole idea of "feeling uptight" probably stems from dysfunction of our Pericardium Meridian bi-laterally AND dysfunction of our Small Intestine meridians, which represent kindness."

Lack of feeling generous? Lack of feeling grateful? Feeling the harshness (unkindness) of the world and people? You're probably going to have tight shoulders.

Checking for healthy direction of flow in these meridians and tracing them if disturbances exist, can be done by college freshmen. It's simple.

We make conditions more pleasant for our heart muscle by healthy flow in our Generosity and Gratitude meridians.

If this sounds new to you, it is. This in an offshoot of the topic of Heart Psychology, begun by Julie Motz in her book *Hands of Life*. The few pages devoted to this topic helped me understand how the heart muscle is only Thumper the rabbit in the original Bambi cartoon movie; it is the organ of drive and real-time interaction with the world. The heart muscle per se is not the organ of pink hearts, flowers and loving--this is the Pericardium. The inner experience of loving is the "pay off" for all the activity and drive of the heart, its comfort and reward.

Because of the need for LOVING and its general absence as a quality in traditional acupuncture, I believe the better name for the Circulation-Sex meridian is the Pericardium Meridian.

Healthy, positive, balanced: Staying aware in the present, enthusiasm, healthy impulse control, appropriate dependency, healthy interest in the outer world. Satiated, tranquil. Healthy playful risk taking; the rejuvenating power of play; healthy play derives some of its pleasure from taking and succeeding at small risks.

Axis of Dysfunction ~ numbing out on passive addictions; on the other hand, flying off the handle in reckless over-activity.

UNDER- pole dysfunction: addicted to numbing out on gloomy, passive addictions to get away from the anxiety of a crisis of identity.

OVER- pole dysfunction: addiction to active, harsh, reckless, sensationalism (hysteria is the old term) to get away from the anxiety of a crisis of identity.

"Anything to reduce [self] awareness"~ *Whisenant*

Whisenant says more on this meridian than any other. His account gives the impression more of his patients had this as their basic imbalance; and, addressing this imbalance did more good for more patients than any other single meridian. In this we can surmise Whisenant speculates Circulation Sex imbalance is somewhat characteristic and emblematic of out-of-balance North Americans. North Americans who are addicted to alternating between over-work and then passive, numbing couch potato activity at home, act out the extremes of the dysfunctional Pericardium Meridian.

The tendency of both under- and overcharge conditions is behavior to reduce internal awareness; in a word: distraction. Switching and swapping addictions is how we stay distracted from what we are authentically thinking-and feeling. Think: Problems with impulse control, paralyzing passions. Think: unwillingness to consider the consequence of past or future actions, distracting ourselves from the "hard work" of thinking-feeling about the consequences of our choices. Think: Drive to keep painful information and unresolved material unconscious.

At one extreme, think, extremely painful memories we wish to reduce awareness of. "Keep those feelings compartmentalized!"

Fear of looking inside, fear of making our own moral evaluations and/or fear of our own self-judgments and Inner Critic. Fear of anything like Truth. Denial, discounting.

Replace genuine feelings with shoulds and oughts. Harsh to others and harsh to self.

Internal "management vs. union" conflicts. If unresolved, over time, this leads to self-sabotage.

Jealousy and sexual tension (not sexual indecision. That goes with kidney meridian).

Other clues to dysfunction: Repressed acute grief. Repressed shock as in PTSD. Broken trust, repressed betrayal. Repressed deep yearning. Sexual transitions at puberty & menopause. Frustrated self-expression.

UNDERcharged expressions of Pericardium

Passive addictions, dulling awareness, numbing out on alcohol, barbiturates and other downers. "Go away and forget it all." Lowers their arousal level. Gloomy (reduced awareness plus stress of repressing and avoiding awareness of consequences).

Repressed identity crisis, passive response to "Who am I?." Regret, remorse, I'm unlovable. Excessive sensory deprivation, emotional withdrawal.

Slavish worship of anything. "Do me, take over for me." Slavish guru worship so as to give over personal responsibility to another. Takes on and adopts an external moral code uncritically (to save themselves from inner examination). Spiritual channeling if from a drive to get yourself out of the way and let someone else take over. "Do me."

UNDER- metaphors & myths: Couch potato. Solitaire addicts, chess addicts. Alcoholics, downer addicts. Followers-worshipers of passive, quietistic cults who abandon their critical thinking skills.

OVERcharged CIRC SEX expressions: Hysteria (common up thru Freud's era but no longer common today). Harsh to others and harsh to self. Acting our identity crisis, over-active response to "Who am I?" Addiction to ACTIVE behaviors, like extreme sports, go all out in sports, use them like a drug. Addiction to first person shooter video games. These are killing simulators, encouraging and validating the answer to all problems is extreme violence, brutality and killing, addicting players players to remove all problems quickly thru force; life as a KillZone video game.

Prefers **activities** which raise and manipulate arousal: over-work, shopaholic behavior, obsessive exercise, making a joke out of everything, sexualizing normal acts and activities. Exaggerated expressions of laughter and seduction (Whisenant). Acting out, tribal dancing of various kinds. Use any of the above like a drug.

Abandon their critical thinking skills going into dangerous activities: Eviel Knievel.

Prefers **drugs and foods** which raise and manipulate arousal: "upper" drugs, caffeine, sugar, hard drugs. Use these as "an activity," excuse them to close friends as "lifestyle choices."

Drug addicts who swap one addiction for another endlessly. Switching and swapping partners, addictions, sensations. Problems with impulse control, with denial, with discounting the feelings of others, with projecting onto close friends, with paralyzing passions and pressures.

Replace genuine feelings with shoulds and oughts. Takes on and adopts an external moral code uncritically to save themselves from deeper inner examination. External moral codes from parents, gurus, churches, fringe politics, drug culture are all fair game.

Metaphors and Myths for OVERcharged CIRC SEX:

Men: The Playboy. Lancelot in the playboy phase: out of touch with his passions because he is bound up with addictive activity.

Oedipus – oblivious, blatant blind spots, oblivious to the consequences of his actions, in the dark about his own actions and their consequences. He deals with his own sins no more gracefully than he dealt with others'. Oedipus puts out his eyes to reduce his conscious awareness. Blatant blind spots. To outsiders his "blindness" is pitiful (*Whisenant* 106-109).

The Joker in Batman: the aggressive thrill seeker, over-stimulated, excessive joking around, constant joking around, addictive joking around. Critical thinking turned self-destructive. The Joker can also stand for an identity crisis in overcharged phase.

The Christopher Lee Dracula movies, especially in "Taste the Blood of Dracula," circa 1975.

Renfrew played by Dwight Frye in the 1931 Bela Lugosi Dracula, hunting flies and eating them.

Women: The Vamp as in the silent movie icon, Theda Bara, also female vampire seductresses.

Madonna the singer, in her early days. Aggressive thrill seeking. Sensationalism.

Guinevere in her fickle, seductive phase, jealous, shallow, histrionic (clinging as histrionics). Likes men fighting fighting over her for her amusement.

Lancelot in the over phase is a playboy, out of touch with his passions because he is bound up with addictive activity and blind to possible negative consequences.

Other Pericardium energy lore

+ Anorexia - *Whisenant* says most addictive behavior stems from circ-sex meridian imbalance; except anorexia, which is stomach meridian. He says don't let anorexics be lumped in with substance abusers. Substance abuse tends to be circ-sex imbalance. Anorexia is a different pattern, a stomach pattern. See stomach meridian section.

+ Affirmations~ for RIGHT meridian: I am generous. For LEFT meridian: I am grateful. For BOTH sides: My body is relaxed and open, Love [from the larger field around my physical body] flows thru me [I am a conduit for loving from a source bigger than my own field of ego].

For RIGHT meridian: I renounce old habits and behaviors no longer aligned with relaxing into Love.

For LEFT meridian: I renounce, let go, release unhealthy attachments number 1, number 2, number 3 ...

-=+ -=+ -=+-=+ -=+ -=+-=+ -=+ -=+

HEART Meridian

Not the pericardium surrounding the heart organ

Fire Yin

T4H muscle: Subscapularis

Healthy headline (positive & balanced): Life-giving to others as you have been given life by others. Generous to self and others, always towards personal balance and contentment; therefore, forgiveness, compassion. Meet life's challenges resiliently, not exhausting self. Self-forgiveness in the personal domain. Flowing with what can and cannot be controlled, towards building healthy, collaborative contentment: how young King Arthur built Camelot.

Inwardly secure; therefore, capacity for appreciation, gratefulness, forgiveness, benevolence, compassion, community-building. "I love you," aligned passion, conviction, loyalty to one's own joy without being egocentric.

Negative emotions absorbed: heartache, broken-hearted, lost passion, emotionally insecure.

Axis of Dysfunction ~ No compassion for self; on the other hand, no compassion for others, only compassion for self.

UNDER- pole Heart dysfunction: Overly selfless as in unlived passion, no compassion for self.

OVER- pole Heart dysfunction: Type A personality. Egocentric, exaggerated personal passion, little compassion for others.

Muscle Metaphors from *T4H 2nd Ed*: Hiding my emotions, keeping all my feelings private, holding onto feelings I need to reveal(undercharge). Revealing my feelings to others appropriately (balance). Receiving too many messages about my life and within my Soul in daily activity (overcharge) (adapted from p 135).

Other UNDERcharged behavior: feeling used, feeling left out, humiliated, unexpressed loving, having no right to self-expression: Not being heard; not being seen. Unlived joy. Boredom, emotionally uncreative, repressed, self-absorbed in a slumped manner, self-protected.

Indecisive, giving up, insecure, inhibited, choked, meekness, humble and modest, always ready to carry out orders from outer authority. Low assertiveness. Overly reserved. Gives in to control of others; gave in to the control of one parent. Caves in to control by others. Needs assertiveness training.

UNDER- metaphors & MYTH: Willy Loman (especially Lee J. Cobb portrayal) in "Death of a Salesman," overwhelming fatigue, fear and dread.

Moses (*Whisenant* 236-238). Charlton Heston's performance as Moses is very much off the historical mark. Moses saw himself as incompetent as a leader. He was famously slow of tongue. Find a more likely representation of both Moses and Pharaoh in Emil Bock's book, Moses. Additional useful resources for the historical Moses are desirable.

Other OVERcharged HEART expressions: chronic activation (always "on"), exhausts self, multi-phase activity. Time urgency. Rigid over-control of as many factors as possible, control at all costs, dictator, iron-clad, hard-hearted. Fear of loss of control, sub- and unconscious hostility and intolerance. Wants to know who's got the power all the time.

OVERcharged HEART MYTH: Pharaoh at the time of Moses. Pharaoh is a hard-hearted dictator. strives to control all aspects of his culture and society even if it leads to wholesale destruction.

Other energetic HEART lore

+ Carol Ritberger observes the heart absorbs different unresolved emotions in each quadrant:

Upper right quadrant - fear (close to throat)

Lower right quadrant - anger (close to liver)

Upper left quadrant - betrayal

Lower left quadrant - sadness (close to spleen)

Holistic Blood Chemistry
http://modernherbaleducation.com/downloads/HolisticBloodChemistry3x.pdf
makes clear the emotional context of high and low cholesterol: High Cholesterol creates difficulty processing emotions, aggressive, demanding, moody, irritable, prone to emotional outbursts.

Low Cholesterol creates holding emotions in, low Serotonin Levels, oxidative stress, Cardiovascular Disease, Heavy Metal Toxicity, elevated cancer risk, high suicide rate.

In other words, very similar to the emotional context of high and low blood pressure.

-=+ -=+ -=+ -=+ -=+ -=+ -=+ -=+ -=+

SMALL INTESTINE Meridian & Organ

Fire Yang

Quadraceps ~ Abdominals

Healthy balanced: Organ ~ Taking in, assimilating and incorporating the good things in life flowing by; giving back smiles and connection. Recognizing good things and taking them in. Flowing, absorbing, easy assimilation.

SI has left and right portions. On left-most 2/5 of small intestine: patient, solitary activity, clear of distracting internal confusions (think Merlin and bookkeepers). On right-most 3/5 of SI, balanced attention to detail, able to see how all small details fit into larger picture, easy travel between details and the large vision (think CEOs like King Arthur).

Meridian ~ Receiving and giving kindnesses. The milk of human kindness learned in healthy mutual bonding between newborns and breast-feeding mothers. Gentleness, nourishment experienced as kindness

Contentment in the heart rests on kindness in the SI as both are fire organs. Unconsciously content; therefore, physical vitality, aliveness, sustainable emotional endurance.

Headline Axis of Dysfunction is kindness~anxiety. Anxiety as overwhelm, as unconscious distraction-confusion, therefore easily misinterpreting the intentions of others. Stress from unknown causes. Dissociation.

Secondary Axis of Dysfunction is Big picture~details. Cares only about the big picture, not the details of life OR cares only about the details, overwhelmed by details, life's big picture escapes them.

Negative emotions absorbed: anxiety, free-floating anxiety, over-excited, unconscious shock, sadness, feeling unappreciated, nervousness, discouraged, unconscious assimilation, unconscious wounds & hurting, abandonment.

UNDER- pole dysfunction: uninvolved in the details of life, cares only about the big picture, wide-tolerant, cant see the trees--only the whole forest, careless about details

OVER- pole dysfunction: Over-responsive to details, close-tolerant, can't see the forest--only the trees, sees only details, careless about the big picture, lacks the big picture, avoids the big picture.

Other emblematic dysfunctions (under-over): Tension with the personal Shadow, shock, sorrow, sadness, nervousness, unconscious wounds and hurting, dread, unresponsive to the world. Feeling lost, abandoned, deserted, forsaken, victimy.

"Nobody speaks clearly to me. Try as I might, I always seem to misunderstand what others are saying" ~ Lonny Jarrett, *Nourishing Destiny*.

Other UNDERcharged behavior: Overwhelmed, bogged down in detail, lose the larger vision; therefore, procrastination, feel trapped by life, unconsciously inhibited, unconsciously unlovable. All things low self-esteem, worthless, shame and personal toxicity.

Digestion, assimilation issues possibly related to inability to assimilate past life experiences. Deprived of nourishment, hungry for warmth, closeness, acceptance, love, safety, intimacy.

A lost & vulnerable child, timid, shy, neglected, forsaken, abandoned. Deeply lonely, deep unconscious grief.

Hidden shame, hidden abuse, hidden regret, hidden guilt, hidden humiliation. Hidden dark secrets, family secrets.

From the outside, easy for others to criticize them; others try to get them organized. What the cerebral does not see is the fear, how gargantuan small tasks appear (Mimi Castellanos). Perfectionism, attached to doing all tasks perfectly (overcharge). Go numb in order not to be bothered by unwelcome thoughts, ideas and habits.

These expressions can be found mixed with manipulation in some individuals.

UNDERcharge Sm. Int. MYTH: Oscar Madison in the "Odd Couple," the "slob." Also Sisyphus, feeling like marriage, job, life is a never-ending task or burden (*Whisenant* 252-260).

Other OVERcharged behavior: obsessive compulsive, perfectionism driven by the thought, "When I become perfect, I will be loved, accepted, etc." Suffers insistent, repetitive ideas and compulsive habits. Obsessed with details. The person's behavior, routines and habits are so repetitive and rigid as to be stereotyped. Can't delegate responsibility. Scrupulous to unreason, perfectionist. Impatient.

OVERcharge MYTH: Felix Unger in the "Odd Couple," the fastidious neatnik (*Whisenant* p 252-260).

UNDERcharge Sm. Int. METAPHOR: Laurel & Hardy: "Nobody speaks clearly to me. Try as I might, I always seem to misunderstand what others are saying."

Whisenant also cites the myth, Psyche & Cupid, for both over & undercharge, in different sections of her myth. One aspect of Whisenant's analysis: "Like the person with a dysfunctional Small Intestine Meridian, Psyche finds herself cut off from mortal humans. In her [overcharged] world of [unrealistic] perfection, there can be no real people because genuine humans are imperfect. They are often dirty; they make mistakes and they feel the whole gamut of emotions: sadness, anger, fear not just [the feelings you want or expect them to feel]" (*Whisenant* 253).

Other energetic SM. INTESTINE lore

+ Matthew Wood says SI is one of the supremely unconscious organs. It is supposed to be, and to remain, unconscious, be design. Villi in the SI have the job of discerning which proteins and nutrients flowing by are safe and beneficial to the whole person and which things flowing by are not safe or not beneficial now.

+ Why does the small intestine meridian appear on the hand, arm, shoulder, face, really far away from the organ? We express kindness with our hands, arms, face, reaching out. Images.google.com has images of "hand of christ." In them you can see the gesture of the healthy small intestine meridian.

+ Because small intestine is naturally unconscious and "out of it" relative to the external world, it relates with the archetype of the absent-minded professor.

+ Merlin's profoundly deep unrequited love for Niume, who betrays him, also expresses the SI's ability to hold onto things unworkable for it for ages and eons.

+ A metaphor for our Habit Body is the "salt grinder at the bottom of the ocean" endlessly grinding out salt. Why? The last instruction the grinder received was to make salt, its last explicit conditioning. It's waiting for a new instruction it trusts.

As the "brain at the other end of our body," SI is perhaps the primary organ of intelligence in our Habit Body. If it is programmed into lack and poverty, it keeps bringing these out--until it receives new programming instructions it believes are trustworthy.

+ As "the brain at the other end of the body." SI is a dimmer mirror reflection of cerebral brain intelligences. SI is as active and unconscious in the south pole of our body as our cerebral brain is active and unconscious in the north pole of our body. Far from being treated as an equal, compared to our cerebral brain, our SI gets no respect.

+ Small Intestine as archetype for dowsing, kinesiology testing and self-testing of all kinds because: What is the small intestine doing all day, 24/7? Each of its little villi "fingers" are poking into a stream of nutrients flowing by, sensing amino acids and other available nutrients, a chemical conversation. We can express it this way. The villi asks itself, "is this nutrient I'm in contact with true for me; or, not true for me?" If the nutrient is "true for me," it is taken into the blood stream and circulated to where it can be used a building block of tissue. If the answer is "not true for me," the nutrient is allowed to slip by.

Dowsing and K-testing of all kinds is nothing more nor less than more conscious versions of this inner self-talk, applying this same self-sensitivity to other decisions and in larger contexts. One common application is, "Is bottle of vitamins X beneficial for me now? True or not true for me?" and, comparing how beneficial bottle of vitamins X is compared to bottle of vitamins, Y.

+ The SI is designed to separate the impure from the pure. Therefore its dysfunction "thesis" can be, "Either I am confused or you are confused" ~ Lonny Jarrett. The chronic misunderstanding of Laurel & Hardy is archetypal here.

Small intestine as repository of psychic genetic material. When I "met" the energetic contents of my own small intestine, I learned two things. I learned we choose the family we choose to embody into not only for the more surfacy mental-emotional karma of mom and dad. Mom and dad help us recap our unresolved issues quickly by their proximity. Up to age seven at least, we also reach out unconditionally to sponge up the unconscious activity of mom and dad as well.

Along this same line, we also choose our family not only for mom and dad; we also choose it for the grandparents, great-grand parents and so on, on both sides of our family. Some ancestral issues are relevant as issues with our mom and dad. Learning how my small intestine issues tracked back primarily to this kind of "psychic genetic" material was an eye-opener for me. This is why very experienced Health Intuitives check ancestry, in one form or another, as one category of unresolved disturbance.

The other thing I learned in correcting my SI is, perhaps more than any other internal organ it is helped by J-R's dictum: Take only the good, the beautiful and the true and leave all the rest to God. This is the job of the SI. In its terms: recognize and take in all nutrients useful to this body at this time. Leave all the rest to the large intestine and the rectum.

Once the healthy expression of the SI is known, unhealthy, dysfunctional expressions are obvious: inability to recognize nutrients, inability to absorb nutrients, inability to match nutrients to the larger body system. These SI dysfunctions may pertain to skinny people unable to gain weight who wish to gain weight.

+ Similarity of stomach & small intestine meridian issues

Both the stomach organ and small intestine organ contribute nerve tissue to the mass of the enteric nervous system (Mimi Castellanos). Their issues are often overlapping. The useful distinction Bruce sees is stomach issues are more sub-conscious while small intestine issues are much more unconscious. Stomach issues are much more available in and thru the inner child. Small intestine issues are far more likely to lack language, images and other reference points.

Mimi says overwhelm is the prime enteric dysfunction; the person cannot see the whole forest because can only see individual trees. Enterics are often frightened into immobility by the big picture. Tasks look gargantuan. They go numb, cannot muster enuf courage to tackle anything. Paperwork, yardwork, taxes, social obligations all go to pot. Pack rat who saves old newspapers.

Whisenant calls obsessive compulsive behavior a strategy to avoid the more gentle, relaxed and non-controlled give and take of healthy social interaction, the "relaxed and non-controlled give and take of healthy social interaction" is perceived as unsafe.

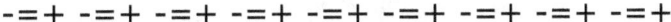

-=+ -=+ -=+ -=+ -=+ -=+ -=+ -=+ -=+

TRIPLE WARMER Meridian

Fire Yang

Teres Minor

Other names: Triple burner, triple heater.

Healthy, positive, balanced: emotional buoyancy, perhaps contented singing. Musical note E, lifting up, living lightly on the Earth, "lightness of being."

Negative emotions absorbed: mood swings, mood disorders, mania & depression, unconscious despair, bi-polar. PTSD.

Axis of Dysfunction ~ heavy depression; on the other hand, exaggerated lightness, mania.

Speculation: Could healthy balanced TW be our antenna for opportunities to be of service to others?

UNDERcharged TW behavior: Despair, despondent, emotional weight, unconscious heaviness, loneliness, feeling exhausted, loss of faith. Emotional fragility, shock, trauma, PTSD, fear of dissolution (check for early life and past life PTSD).

+ Chloe Faith Wordsworth on Under-charged TW

I am lonely and too isolated. I belong to no group nor community. I feel excluded. Too many of my problems seem overwhelming, disproportionately large. I am uncomfortable in group situations. Just the thought of speaking in public triggers me.

Balanced TW: I am a source of life-giving warmth. I create safe, healthy atmosphere between people. I am warm, loving and charming. I draw people together through my human warmth and interest. I naturally create healthy webs and networks between people and groups. I draw people together for relaxation, fun and connection. From: *Transforming Five Element and Meridian Patterns with Resonance Repatterning* (2012)

Two kinds of depression ~ *Whisenant* talks about depression as meridian phenomena. He talks about two kinds of depression related to TW, low adrenal and low thyroid. Neither of these has the more active, raging depression expressed in liver-GB depression. Low adrenal depression is exhaustion & low energy. Low thyroid depression is brooding and morbid. See Thyroid below, "nothing for me."

In TW depression, too much energy is held too high in the body and in the head (overcharge). Even if not intellectual, relies on thinking; the person relies very much on the cerebral nervous system. These people are killer players at trivial pursuit" (*Whisenant*). May subscribe to the "Cult of the New," the "new, new thing" (Kevin Kelly of Wired magazine), uncritically adopting the new as an end in itself. See also spleen overcharge on uncritical acceptance.

Consequently In TW depression, lower body is under-charged. Common symptoms of lower-body undercharge include knee problems and low body temp. "Palms face backwards. Slumping posture. Sensitive to cold" (*Whisenant*). Knee problems as metaphor ~ When too much body energy is centered in and around the head, energy is too high in the body, lower half is undernourished.

UNDER-TW metaphors & myths: Daedalus, the master craftsman/detective, the quiet, subversive radical (*Whisenant* 128-133). Absent-minded professor, ideas are over-thought. High tolerance for physical disorder.

Unwillingness to bring their higher self in contact with the earth thru kneeling (*Msgs. from the Body*).

OVER-charge TW expressions: Manic is the classic overcharge expression. Over-creating. High body temp. Over-functioning of thyroid and adrenals, agitated, restless. Live dangerously, thoughtless for their own safety, live close to the edge. Death wish? Palms may face forward. Sanpaku.

OVER-TW metaphors & myths: Icarus, the manic, flying too high and getting burned, reckless, live dangerously, thoughtless for own safety (*Whisenant* 128-133).

Other energetic Triple Warmer lore

+ Possible to have PTSD and/or manic-depressive episodes coming up from past lives. If this tests "yes," count how many; ask for your own Higher Guidance to stack them in priority, priority episode on top or in front. Bring in peace.

+ Triple what exactly?

The original exact implication of "triple" in Triple Warmer is apparently lost (David Feinstein). Current consensus appears to have shifted in the last ten years towards viewing TW as our stress response. TW points to thyroid and amygdalae. 5,000 years ago when meridians were named, another unknown torso organ was implicated. Humanity seems to have evolved so this third function is now higher in body?

Without mentioning any associated single organ, in his *Nourishing Destiny, The Inner Tradition of Chinese Medicine* (1998) Lonny Jarrett discusses two meridians, Circ-Sex (Pericardium Meridian, Heart Protector Meridian); and, Triple Warmer. These two as shock absorbers for heart muscle activity:

TW especially provides an outermost defense system, dispersing or absorbing shock and trauma; keeping unnecessary mood swings outside and away from disturbing the necessary, steady vortexing of vitality into the blood our heart muscle provides.

Jarrett describes Pericardium Meridian as protecting our emotional heart. Thru its romantic, heart-filled, heartfelt feelings, the health of our Loving Heart Center, in front of breastbone, our feeling heart forces is nourished and protected. Jarret implies TW works with Pericardium meridian to screen inappropriate external stimulus before it is allowed all the way into our inner sanctum, into intimate contact with both our physical and emotional heart.

Healthy function of TW, ". . .receives blows meant for the heart. . . It is paramount for stopping potentially damaging insults to our heart at outer layers of defense. If threat or invasion ever reaches the castle gates, a good part of the damage may have already been done. . . In order to fulfill this function, the triple heater maintains constant connection with every relevant aspect of our surroundings" (Jarrett 218).

Jarrett points to infancy and childhood, where the delicate and vulnerable emotional heart of a child needs and requires protection. Adult caregivers perform this protective function until the infant develops its own healthy immune responses and Triple Warmer function to deal with harsh environments.

If over-protection of a child's heart continues too far into adulthood, there can be hyper-sensitivity to impacts from other persons. This can dull awareness of a child's love; or, from a loving and appropriate suitor. Over-charged TW permits hyper-sensitivity to environmental toxins. A healthy adult with good Self-leadership is more resourceful. Every stimulus need not be treated as an attack. Over-reacting is an infant's response to harsh elements of 3D life.

Imbalanced TW, over or under, seems to track back to unresolved memories of shock, trauma, PTSD trapped in the body. Check thyroid, amygdalae (bilateral), and hypothalamus. These can all affect TW. Secondarily check adrenals and heart. Which issues predominate in an individual: thyroid, hypothalamus or adrenal issues--is individual. Hence, the usefulness of testing the client's immune system directly.

Thyroid psychology

Mimi Castellanos (BravoCoop.com, HealthyEnergetics.net) says when the thyroid is out of balance it goes towards either ALL ABOUT ME (over-charge) or goes towards NOTHING FOR ME (under-charge). Very common to flit back and forth between these two. Very common to have left or right "wing" of thyroid stuck in one or the other. Check!

Thyroid weakness is aggravated by weak Governing Vessel, our meridian of healthy self-concept. Over-charged GV suggests arrogance, too-high self-concept, grand narcissism. Low GV suggests absence of healthy self-concept, potential to feel like a "lowly worm." Most elegant way to clear is to build up the weak under-charge. Then toxic over-charge calms down. It was simply compensating for the under-charge.

Energetic thyroid lore

Thyroid can be imagined as a bow-tie shape, with both sides, both triangles the same size and in balance. A bow-tie images a balanced thyroid. In clients, we find the right and left sides of the thyroid can be different sized, Check if one side is over-charged and the other side undercharged.

+ Hypothroidism type 2 ~ Doctors Jerry Tennant and Mark Starr, both recommended by Matt Stone, agree Broda Barnes was correct: A huge fraction of people have low metabolic rate brought about by low iodine support for thyroid, thyroid damage, or both. This used to be very common. Now sub-clinical levels are even more widespread yet undiagnosed because of the narrow range of thyroid markers targeted in blood tests.

Thyroid affects even body build. Low thyroid can cause children to grow too tall too quickly (current author's body expression) or cause children to grow short and squat. This suggests the topic of thyroid metabolism is only superficially addressed by conventional docs. Tennant and Starr, building on Broda share current Best Practices.

Some people say lack of half moons on fingernails signals absence of iodine. I can find no contradiction to this. Lugol's iodine, liquid, works well. If too challenging, work with iodine capsules. Lugol's is now available in inexpensive dried, dehydrated capsules.

Hypothalamus psychology

As they say, hypothalamus appears to be fight, flight, or freeze.

Amygdalae psychology

What does triple warmer perceive? It perceive threats and shocks from outside, coming towards the body. TW is YANG Fire. "... it networks the energies of all the meridians to counter an invader. ... Triple warmer prepares the body for war! - Donna Eden. It's response to perceived threats and shocks is always going to be YANG.

The two amygdalae, inside either side of the temples, are commonly associated with fright. Bruce also associates them with PTSD, "shock and awe." They may also be associated with "deer in the headlights" behavior as when deer are overloaded, they get "frozen."

+ The "little me" dilemma: Note how thyroid and hypothalamus dysfunction, both in the upper part of the body, are both "about me," me, me , me. Either "all about me" or "nothing at all for me." Watch out for the danger of boredom. It competes with being of service to others. Our small "s" self (ego) is capable of going round and around, back and forth between "all about me" and "nothing for me" in endless reactivity, forgetting to be of service where clear to do so.

Suggestion: ask for a spiritual perspective. "What is Spirit trying to create thru me?" and, "How can Spirit flow more down, thru me, and out to other people, at this time?" This connects the small "s" self with our capital "S" Self. Shift perspective from "little me" to a larger social context of the highest good for all concerned. Such questions can lead to actions which become a source of peace for TW meridian.

Passengers in a moving car, especially passengers riding in the front passenger seat ~ Perception of threat ~ If as passenger, the car we are in approaches the back of a big bus faster than we feel is safe; and, we perceive our driver isnt slowing down soon enuf, we involuntarily stomp down on the floor where the car brake pedal would be--if we were driving. We may also put our hands up in front of our face, bracing for impact. This is amygdala, TW or some combination "doing its job," responding to perception of threat.

Donna Eden: Sedating TW flushing the meridian by hand

Donna Eden's technique of sedating TW by running the meridian backwards by hand is classic. It can be found in her original Energy Medicine volume and online.

+ Triple Warmer-Spleen pattern

Donna Eden and EFT self-healers have done a lot of work here. You can Google the topic: "Triple Warmer-Spleen pattern" to see many pages. A report from a class of Donna Eden's:

The Triple Warmer turns on a fight/flight stress response when it feels threatened. Unfortunately, in our culture, Triple Warmer often turns on [overcharge] when it doesn't need to, treating anything it doesn't understand as an enemy [including relatively minor disturbances such as overhead fluorescent lighting].

When Triple Warmer goes into overdrive, it first pulls energy from the Spleen meridian... and then from every other meridian, affecting the Heart meridian last.

I remember being at an Energy Medicine intensive where the audience was asking Donna Eden the cause of different conditions... and she kept answering "Triple Warmer Spleen imbalance." Asked about the cause of food allergies, or allergies in general, Donna answered, Triple Warmer Spleen imbalance. Fear and depression? Triple Warmer Spleen imbalance. Blood sugar problem? Candida? Triple Warmer Spleen imbalance. MS? Arthritis? Shingles?: Triple Warmer Spleen imbalance. Thyroid problems? Chronic fatigue syndrome? Triple Warmer Spleen imbalance. Sore throat? Any sort of infection? Triple Warmer Spleen imbalance. Stress, pain or tension? Triple Warmer Spleen imbalance. Overindulging in anything, including compulsive overeating? Triple Warmer Spleen imbalance. How about hot flashes? Hormonal changes? You got it Triple Warmer Spleen imbalance.

I began to better understand how Triple Warmer – Spleen energy imbalances are behind many problems -- Gwenn Bonnel
http://www.tapintoheaven.com/newsletters/Gamut

-=+ -=+ -=+-=+ -=+ -=+-=+ -=+ -=+

A few words on the Sprouting (wood) element

Confusing me and several generations of Western students, the "wood" element characterization naturally links with "lumber."

A better characterization is "sprouting energy," the energy permitting new plants to break thru concrete. This energy is on display especially in all sprouts, especially young wheat grass shoots. Lonny Jarrett points to bamboo before, during and after a windstorm as demonstrating directionality about its own growth, emptiness of ego (bamboo is hollow) and resilience after being man-handled by life.

When we stopped being farmers, we also lost our sense of what wood meant in the TCM sense. This is how "dolphin energy" replaced "wood" to represent resilience and joy, an unstoppable forward drive.

The dysfunctional axis of sprouting wood energy appears to be

Overcharge - pushing the river, pushyness, willfulness

Undercharge - pathetic contraction, "my get up and go, got up and left." The undercharge is easy to mistake for left side spleen-pancreas undercharge—and—the two often go together because both are on the level of "feeling."

-=+ -=+ -=+ -=+ -=+ -=+ -=+ -=+

LIVER Meridian

SPROUTING wood Yin

Pectoralis Major Sternal ~ Rhomboids

Healthy, positive, balanced: The open, healthy optimism and enthusiasm of teenage years, inspirational youthful vitality and resilience. Shouting for joy, joy bubbling up especially in children and teens. Openness to other's point of view, works well with others. Healthy assertion of own views, mental flexibility. Pliant to personal changes.

Forbearance, polite self-assertiveness, motivation. Trusting. Composed emotionally, especially at home. Ready to forgive & forget difficulties. Orderly movement between energy and matter. Conscientious, reliable.

Negative psychology absorbed: unfocused wrath, frustration, projection and transference of emotions and motivations, onto others.

Axis of Dysfunction ~ emotional contraction, homelessness, also utter despair; on the other hand, raging like a storm at sea.

Main UNDER- pole dysfunction: Depressed, overcome by feelings of worthlessness, low self-esteem. Pathetic contraction of all expansive forces, as in many homeless persons.

Main OVER- pole dysfunction: thru their behavior, demands to be the center of attention, raging like a storm at sea towards anyone and everyone present, due to frustration and angst (enteric dominant). Insolence, intellectually arrogant (cerebral dominant).

Other main emblematic dysfunctions: Scatter, doing too much, allows, promotes and creates distractions. Emotional outbursts at home. "Full of enthusiasm, Lancelot jumps on his horse and rides off in all directions at once."

Enthusiasm as an end in itself, "bigger is better, more is better." Over-achieving (see also kidney overcharge).

Archie Bunker, played by Carol O'Connor in All In the Family, the father of "Meathead," circa 1980s TV. Chronic foul temper, short temper, shouting, anger, blaming, obnoxious. This is the diffuse discernment power of the liver turned both outward and negative. Loud aggressive stance masks pain and sorrow not fully felt. Unable to find resolution. Unacknowledged deeper feelings. Dispirited

Uncategorized imbalances: Liver organ-meridian imbalances are not conscious; they are primarily SUBconscious, in our feeling zone. Hence, the word "unexamined:"

Unexamined, unresolved feelings

Contentious for no reason

Unexamined frustration, jealousy

Unexamined self-sabotage

Unexamined discontentment & dissatisfaction

Unexamined toxicity affecting self & others

Unexplained dizziness

Irrationality; specifically, inability to connect thoughts with feelings and feelings with thoughts.

Frustrated, discontented, dissatisfied because cannot achieve clarity on feelings. This is frequently diagnosed due to cultural blind spots of parents and teachers about converting feelings into language; and therefore, interpreting feelings to the thinking mind.

Toxic behavior loops, especially if audible as whining and complaining about how bad things are and how they don't get better. If a toxic loop tests as present, ask for the depth of the loop: conscious, subconscious, unconscious. It may be repetition of dysfunctional family history, cultural traditions, etc. Then, ask the Light to interrupt it for the highest good (Mimi).

Other UNDERcharged LIVER expressions: Loss of physical and emotional stamina due to suppressed liver function.

Feeling unacknowledged. co-dependent because feelings of low self-esteem color every decision and action, looks for clarity on self from the outside, from others. Unable to find resolution. Withholding all feelings as has no clarity on them. Dispirited

Whining and complaining, ineffectual complaints. Whisenant says complaining is like bragging about how much one can suffer. Relates to Caroline Myss's topic of Why People Don't Heal and "woundology," having an ailment to talk about is better than having nothing at all to talk about. Anger is more diffuse, not smart bomb anger (gall bladder), less directed towards a target. Complaining as a smoke screen to avoid dealing with the pain of the original target person. Ineffectual complaints.

Lack of foresight and planning. Travels round and around in feelings of low self-esteem, stuck in the gut brain, stuck in feelings. Unable to rise up into clarity and perspective on own feelings. Unable to match feelings with thoughts in a healthy, balanced dance.

Anger blocked by fear. Unwillingness to face the real causes of angry feelings, need to cultivate sensitivity to unfinished grief and sadness. Need to shout, need for cathartic release. Tennis racket work can be useful.

Crying for "no reason," as evidence of inability to match thoughts with feelings. Irrationality. May feel they do not have permission to match thoughts up with feelings, per mom or dad.

Numb to toxic elements, toxic emotions, toxic persons and environmental toxins, suffer toxic people and environments in silence (liver is the main detoxer of the body).

UNDERcharged Liver myth: Epimetheius, brother or Prometheus. Epimetheius is the Underachiever, the faithful, but castrated lieutenant, incapable of taking his own decisive action, incapable of standing up for self (Whisenant 156-162).

Other OVERcharged LIVER behavior: Diffuse out of control anger; unyielding, forceful, short temper. Willfulness & forcefulness for its own sake. Change for change's sake (to relieve frustration). Dizziness, suddenly failing vision.

OVERcharged LIVER myth: Prometheus - obstinately standing alone, intellectually arrogant, defiant, partly rebellious. He is the archetype of being stuck in the cerebral brain unable to dance, to "balance and swing" in a healthy way with his opposite, feelings. Arrogant and complex, even when he wishes not to be. Bright, crafty, even conniving. His fellow Greek gods perceive Prometheus as insolent and overstepping his boundaries and authority, His equals see him as obstinate, standing alone and in opposition, insolent. He upsets the gods three times. His final sentence is to be chained to a rock with an eagle eating his (excessive) liver out daily (*Whisenant* 158-162).

Other energetic LIVER lore

Liver attacking Spleen ~ Generating Controlling Overacting Insulting Cycles in TCM five elements

In Western TCM webpages, the idea of hollow organs (YANG) and solid organs (yin) has great prominence, perhaps to the point of distorting valuable TCM wisdom.

Mr. Google has 748 results for "Regulate and Harmonize the Liver and Spleen"

Mr. Google has 348 results for "liver attacking spleen"

Liver as a solid *yin* organ can obscure three other equally valid TCM views of the Five Elements, the Controlling Cycle, Overacting Cycle and Insulting Cycle.

Control (Ke) Cycle ~ When this works in a healthy way, it functions in the way an understanding grandparent often has more and better influence over an unruly child than the parents do.

When the Control (Ke) Cycle influence is OVERcharged, it becomes the (Destruction, Ke) Cycle. The grandparent organ has too much influence and control over the child organ. This disorder of the Destruction (Ke) Cycle is also called the Overacting (Cheng) Cycle.

> Imbalance within the Control/Ke Cycle can create what is called the Overacting (Cheng) Cycle: an instance in which the "grandmother" element, instead of beneficially "controlling" the grandchild, damages the grandchild element by exerting an inappropriate amount of control, i.e. they "overact" upon that element (citation follows second quote).

The "war within" and "Liver attacking Spleen" are useful metaphors for these dysfunctions.

Its crucial here to bring this into Feeling terms. If Liver is OVERcharged, how does stomach, pancreas, spleen feel?

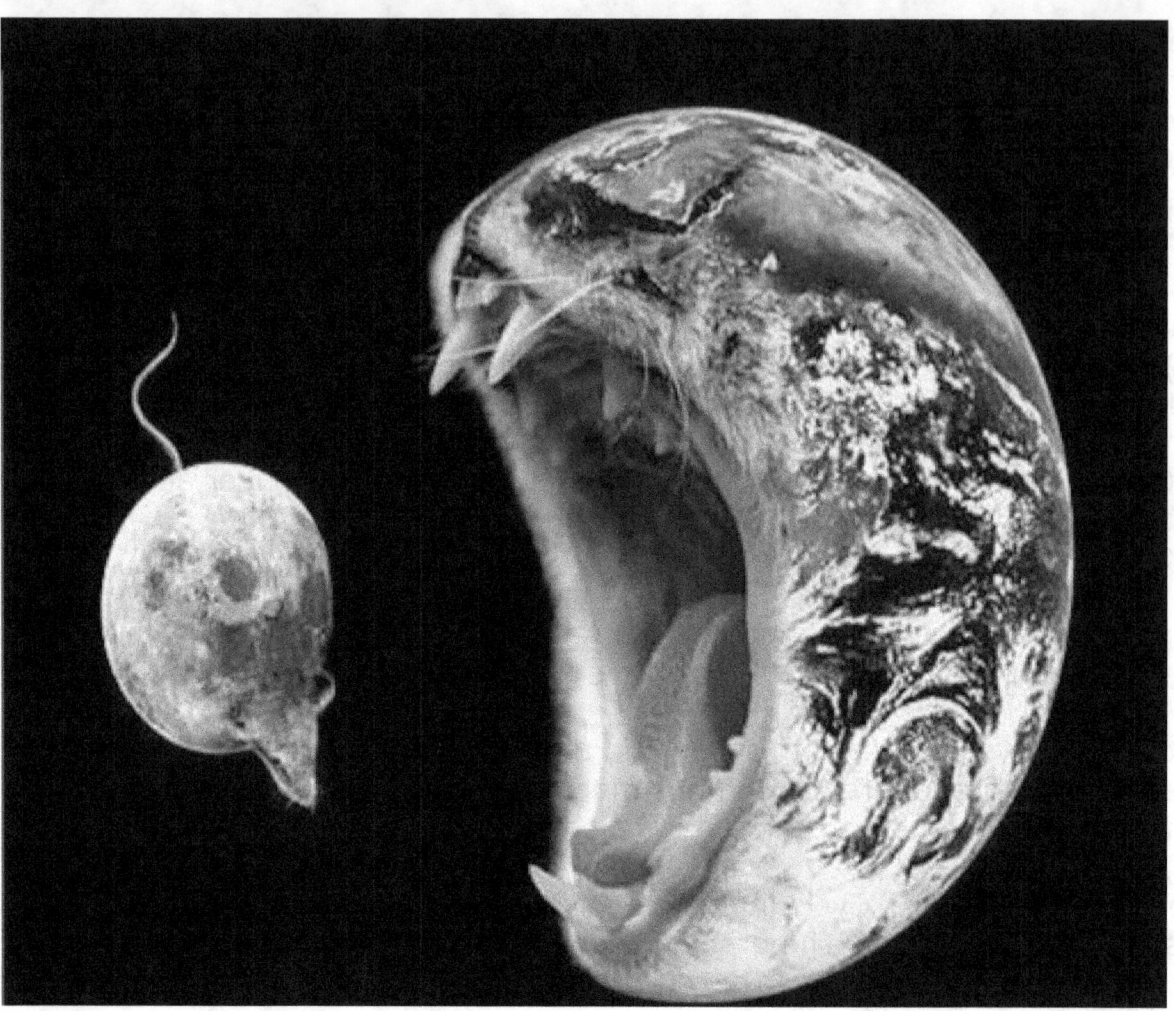

dg- cat and moon-mouse

In the Punch & Judy metaphor, the above covers the Liver side using a stick on the left side. Left side hitting back is covered in the Insulting (Wu) Cycle]

> The Insulting/Wu Cycle represents another instance of unbalanced Control/Ke Cycle functioning. This happens when the "grandchild" element, instead of being beneficially controlled by the "grandmother," turns the grandmother's force back upon itself, hence "insulting" the attempt to control it.
>
> Overacting and Insulting cycles represent imbalanced, disharmonious functions of the Five Element System. Used diagnostically, symptoms of overacting or insulting cycles can provide important feedback, allowing an acupuncturist or Qigong practitioner to intervene in a way to return the system to its balanced Generation & Control Cycle functioning.

Reninger, Elizabeth. "Five Element Dance of Creation (Sheng) & Control (Ke)." Learn Religions, Feb. 8, 2021, LearnReligions.com/five-element-generating-sheng-and-control-ke-cycles-3183168

I believe the above suggests the therapeutic insight of hollow organs (YANG) and solid organs (*yin*) is subordinate to these cycles. It also clarifies "liver attacking spleen."

I believe the above makes the correct connections between the "war within" of all autoimmune disorders and TCM wisdom.

+ Medical Intuitive, Carol Ritberger, observes the liver absorbs different unresolved emotions in each quadrant:

Upper right quadrant - anger

Lower right quadrant - guilt

Upper left quadrant - resentment (closer to spleen)

Lower left quadrant - shame (close to small intestine)

lower right – guilt; lower left – shame (Carol Ritberger).

+ Liver music ~ undercharge is related to music in the minor chord, classically associated with the mood of victimhood. Liver overcharge and bladder meridian overcharge are music in the mood of the third, Souza bands marches, etc.

+ Lancelot-liver connection. In the Inner Court book the liver-Lancelot connection is spelled out in some detail. The short version is both Lancelot in Arthurian Legend and our liver share an obsession with self-purification. Ever hear of "cleanliness is next to godliness"? Liver holds our motivation to purge one's self of guilt and shame. Careful, too many liver cleanses can stress the liver.

The same as everywhere else in our psyche, our liver is prone to carry old stories. Do you enjoy creative visualizations? These old tales can often be seen imaginatively by looking at the back and bottom of your own liver. If you find old stories there, simply ask for the Light of your own Higher Guidance to be your Partner, to clear out all stories no longer necesaary or useful to you now.

Lancelot-liver also share the tendencies to scatter their energies; i.e. alcohol, become distracted, do too much, driven, to over-achieve to compensate for low self-esteem, to jump on his horse and ride off in all directions at once.

Left to himself, Lancelot will worship Enthusiasm as an end in itself. He only functions fully in alignment with the more mature ideals of Arthur, Merlin and Guinever.

+ Liver & spleen as emotional filters

In the enteric nervous system, liver and spleen filter unresolved emotions circulating in the energetic body. Unresolved disturbances settle in the energetic body like "Jello 1-2-3," in layers. If these are left unresolved, new ones come in on top, compress the old ones, until you have an energetic structure analogous to stratified deposits of limestone, seen in raised sea bottom rock--and just as inaccessible (hard to reach). These can be accessed thru kinesiology testing; then, cleared by any of several actions of the soul; most easily, thru forgiveness.

+ The liver-eyes connection

In the liver, seeing and feeling are the same: feeling = seeing = feeling = emotional truth. We see what we feel and we feel what we see. If we stop doing either, we our out of touch with the truth our liver is capable of.

Weak eyes, visual disturbances, cannot use eyes for long periods of time, is classically associated with liver dysfunction. Related to dizziness, another classic liver symptom, better termed, emotional vertigo.

When our emotions are suppressed and repressed, they are pushed down into the subconscious and finally into the unconscious. We become blind to how we feel about things, blind to our own feelings. The healing direction is always to increase willingness to heal; in this case, willingness to see how you feel about yourself, other people, the world, and God.

+ Liver as karmic flywheel. The liver is our largest internal organ. If our body was an engine, the liver is the metabolic and feeling Flywheel, establishing and preserving the momentum and direction of our life. This is most obvious in children prior to puberty. Underlying this is, prior momentum, over and under, from prior existences. Liver is a main organ of karmic continuity, of old ego-stories, happy, angry--whatever quality you embraced and held onto on your emotional roller-coaster ride. Spleen and heart can equally be karmic flywheels.

As in any running engine, it's not healthy to stop the flywheel. If you do, the machine stops running and turns off.

Various liver de-toxes can be beneficial, apple fasts, green smoothies, milk thistle, etc. A deeper level is old ego stories which need clearning out, which may be holding you back. Cleaning your liver of old stories can improve your physical eyesight by releasing unconscious tension.

A good way to approach changing the liver is tolerance, patience and gradualness. Incorporate upgrades without the flywheel slowing down or stopping. A focus on acts of service done with love helps. NOT overextending ourselves to meet others' needs helps. Healthy service counteracts old dysfunctional ego stories of all kinds.

Redeeming the liver from its old stories, myths and role models is a journey. Do I want to live pushed from behind by my old stories? Or do I want to live pulled forward by all the good in my life?

Old habits and stories in the liver will always be familiar and easy to go back to.

+ Liver as the seat of drama ~ Without a workable method to connect with and process Our Inner Game of Life, the Liver, the Child, will turn towards external drama. Why? Without a workable way to process issues internally, unresolved issues will try to resolve themselves thru external drama with whomever is nearly and available. Also, if stories of our past are brighter than stories of our future, our unconscious and our liver will keep looking back towards the past. Our old stories pull us back if we do not have forward momentum into our next creative acts of service to self and for others. So service is healthy therapy for the liver. See also, the Quest for the Holy Grail in Arthurian legend as metaphor for service.

+ TCM clarification: 5,000 year ago, TCM called the liver "the General." However 5,000 years ago the human being was not constituted precisely as we are today. See Rudolf Steiner on this topic. 5,000 years ago, the human being functioned much more out of the gut brain, much less so from the cerebral brain (head brain, hemispheres plus lateral spinal nerves). In the West at least, since the mid-1800s, the cerebral brain has come into its own, has become the locus of control much more fully. The function of "the General," as so vividly expressed by Douglas McArthur, etc, is now called "executive ability." It lives primarily in the left front brain quadrant, represented by King Arthur. To Learn More, *Inner Family + Inner Court; The Four Archetypes of Our Gut and Head.*

-=+ -=+ -=+ -=+ -=+ -=+ -=+ -=+

GALL BLADDER Meridian

Sprouting (wood) Yang

Anterior Deltoid ~ Popliteus

Positive, balanced gall bladder expressions are greatly benefitted by adding the modifying adjective "healthy:" healthy concentration, healthy rhythm, healthy persistence, healthy responsibility.

In general: Self-esteem in making workable choices-decisions in my life, self-esteem in setting and achieving healthy goals. Self-esteem concentrating our energies to make the right decision, at the right, time for the right reason.

Note ~ Both liver and GB can project their focus, imagining one's focus external to self. When negative, "projecting" looks like:

- blaming others and perpetrators,

- identifying external targets,

- scapegoating,

- projecting responsibility-accountability onto perceived enemies.

When mixed with fantasy: making up targets to project responsibility-accountability onto; for example, the Red Scare of the 1950s and Post 9/11 2001 and conspiracy theories which mix both truth and falsehood.

Axis of Dysfunction ~ An axis of "Clear/Confused" seems possible. In the positive, persisting *rhythmically* towards positive, balanced goals: Concentrating our self; and when the time is ripe, taking decisive action. Healthy un-selfconscious action, absence of self-doubt (absence of negative concentration). Defusing conflict & useless polarity. Unsuspecting of hostility from others.

In the negative, confused on how and when to make choices and decisions, internal concentration on a negative focus, negative outbursts of negative action, revenge.

UNDER- pole GB dysfunction: Indecision in personal affairs, "I can't make up my mind!" can't make a personal decision. Unconscious self-doubt. Avoiding action, avoiding commitment; especially, in getting your own needs met,

"I am indecisive about myself." GB has a time polarity of *Fearless* about the future; or, *Fearful* about the future (From Bob Cooley, https://www.thegeniusofflexibility.com/training-archive/gall-bladder).

This can be viewed as an axis of dysfunction: on one end, obsessed about the future, global future, future of humanity. On the other end, "No future for me; I have no future; I see no future for me."

OVER-pole dysfunction: Over-deciding, intolerance. "Get outta my way, you jerk!" Fault finding in other people (classic). Fault finding in your self, out-of-control Inner Critic. Over-responsibility, perpetuating responsibility past its time. Over-concentrating, all your eggs in one conceptual basket.

Over-pole dysfunctions all have to do with over-persistence and lack of rhythmic efforts; including, negativity persisting beyond all practical use. One or both forms of overcharge can be present: pride, certain forms of arrogance, Mr. Know It All. On the other hand: resentment.

Other over-persisting: over-thinking yet unable to discharge, making mountains out of mole hills, especially when obstacles confront personal desires. Overblown polarity with others, imagining and exaggerating the opposition of others. Unwillingness to examine internal contradictions. Unresolved forgiveness issues. These are all unhealthy persistence.

Other UNDERcharged GB expressions: Feeling wronged, feeling there has been a great injustice-but gives up; therefore, futility & resentment in the victim role. Resignation, futility. Lack of power issues. Self-pity, feeling second-best in comparison to another. Needs more spontaneity and self assertion.

"Relationship-shut-down, They don't trust love, have had a history of deeply disappointing relationships. Socially insulated and isolated. Have retreated into themselves, into a state of sad solitude and loneliness (p. 255, *Messages from the Body*, Michael Lincoln, TalkingHearts.net).

Imagined enemies will pour in if defenses are let down. Defeated before I begin due to insufficient personal power, therefore, little likelihood of winning.

Boredom when follow-thru on own goals goes awry or goes off track (form of giving up on self), passivity, humility. Absence of sufficient polarity, lack of adequate distinctions, lack of healthy personal direction, often a part of teenage angst which can continue into 20s or longer.

UNDER- GB metaphors & myths: Tragedy of Macbeth. He feels defeated before he begins, due to insufficient personal power. Therefore: I have little likelihood of winning. Imagined enemies will pour in if I let down my defenses. Macbeth makes distinctions but they are all unhealthy and negative ones.

Macbeth is a picture of victimhood and duality. He can't make decisions and ends up a martyr to his own negative choices; therefore, resignation and futility. Feeling wronged, feeling there has been a great injustice; therefore, resentment in the victimhood role. Needs more spontaneity and self assertion (*Whisenant* 143).

Other OVERcharged GB expressions: The revenge motif used in the plots of 80% of all action movies. Very specific resentments. Stirred up about being wronged, feeling there has been a great injustice and angry the target perpetrator. Unable to discharge the build-up. Vindictiveness.

Over-doing anger where asking nicely would do the job equally well, using a hot knife to cut warm butter. (Rage and frustration per se are liver not GB.)

Unwillingness to share power (an expression of the Establishment 1%?) Impatience, false pride, self-righteousness, overblown polarity with others, mentally two-dimensional, black and white thinking. Manipulative. Bitter, unforgiving, "sore winners" syndrome of "I'm entitled--you're not.

Brutal and or morbid language (Whisenant).

OVER-charged GB myths and metaphors: Lady Macbeth. Specific resentments and angers. Invents imagined enemies, invents polarities where none exist. Sees opposition and adversity everywhere. Imagined grievances and unnecessary rage arise from not viewing situations calmly from varied perspectives, lack of perspective, lack of walking a mile in your adversary's shoes. Vindictive, unwillingness to share power with others.

Lady Macbeth over-creates conscious choices. Over-intensity of conscious and deliberate expression. Feels wronged, feeling there has been a great injustice and angry about it; therefore, resentment, leading to taking on the persecutor role. All moderation is lost, leading to insanity.

Other energetic GB lore

+ Like Bladder meridian, people have the tendency to disturb the flow by trying to pull energy UP the body and concentrate energy in the head (to help them think, they suppose). Many forms of this negative concentration.

+ While GB primarily has to do with concentrating our forces, Bertrand Babinet adds GB also has to do with choice. The GB has a decision to make, when to dump its sac of concentrated bile into the duodenum—but—when to dump? There is no perfect time. So making a choice is always problematic for our friend the gall bladder: when to hold back, when to relax and let go.

GB Overcharge: choosing too forcefully, making too many choices too quickly; hence, intolerance, etc.

GB Undercharge: self-doubt, uncertainty, making too few deliberate choices, hesitancy. Possibly: I can't, I can't, I can't.

+ Speculation: connection between ENTJ and GB meridian In MBTI, the positive traits of an ENTJ are assertive, outspoken, confident, outgoing, energetic, charismatic, fair-minded, not affected by conflict or criticism. The negative traits of ENTJ include appearing argumentative, confrontational, insensitive, intimidating, controlling. They give the impression of overwhelming force, overwhelming one's foes.

The positive and negative traits of ENTJs seem to correlate highly with the over and/or under conditions of the GB.

+ Liver & Gall Bladder as Pirates and Ninjas ~ Some readers will know the internet has a big topic of which is better, pirates or ninjas? I'm waiting for the movies Pirates vs. Ninjas to address this impossible question because both liver and gall bladder are God-given.

Pirate expression is big and loud; they blow up whole ships and think it's fun, "Avast!" and "Ahoy, me hearties!" and "Shiver me timbers!" They THROW THEMSELVES BODILY into battle with reckless abandon, heedless of danger to life and limb, INTOXICATED with the thrill of battle. They live for excitement and action.

Ninja expression is the dark, quiet, the silent killer. Where the Pirate shoots a loud blunderbuss at anything moving, you never hear the ninja until he uses a silent swift sword. The Ninja is not extravagant in his displeasure; no, he has a small piece of paper with a short list of clearly named individuals who must die, who are marked for assassination; preferably, secretly, stealthily with only a red glove left at the scene of the crime as an inarticulate "signature."

Pirates also have a parrot on their shoulder. What does the parrot do? He uses foul language to pointedly SNIPE at his intended targets, targets the Pirate claims he consciously intends not to injure and has only good intentions towards.

The foul mouthed parrot makes pointed comments on your specific facial features, sexual anatomy and preferences, the specific details of sexual relations and habits of your mother and father, the more caustic and incendiary in nature, the better. The parrot's comments are designed to provoke and antagonize but not to prompt direct physical retaliation; at least, so the Pirate thinks. The remarks are like a TIME BOMB sent thru the mail. It only explodes when its target shakes the box.

Here the Pirate represents the liver and his parrot represents the dysfunctional Gall Bladder.

+ GALL BLADDER anger as "smart bomb" anger

Smart-bomb anger wishes to devastate its target. Anger is directed at a specific target (Mimi).

Only with Gall Bladder can liver's power be put behind devastatingly accurate, cutting remarks of the shrewish wife, discerning and pointing out the most demeaning characteristics of others. Women who bust the balls of men thru "mouth surgery." No male version comes to mind but see Archie Bunker in Liver Meridian.

Blaming, projecting onto others, especially projecting personal failure onto others and into the environment. "Just get the heck out of the way already, will you!?" Want to eliminate problems, try to make problems go away as opposed to give and take of negotiating issues. Responds well to cathartic work: tennis racket on bed. Heart meridian over-control is "control every detail." GB control is just get the obstacle out of the way.

+ Paint-roller technique ~ Because your GB meridians are wholly on left and right sides of your body, it's possible to access them by picturing one whole side of your body or the other. If the GB meridian on a side is running backwards, that is UP, imagine a hand paint roller and a pan of paint. Pick a color you wish. In your imagination, roll down the entire right side of your body with your desired color. Unless you are "flushing" the meridian, start rolling from the head and go down towards the feet. This re-trains your Habit Body to flow your energy back into healthy direction of flow. Do the same for the other side. Tomorrow see if the color wants to stay the same or change.

+ GB meridian and shoulder-knee problems - Total Body Management (TBM) has the insight that GB meridian is involved in any and all knee, elbow, wrist and shoulder problems, the sides of the body. For more on the distinct yang quality of the right side of the body and *yin* quality of the left side of the body, see the *The NEW Energy Anatomy.*

+ *Whisenant's* case study of healing GB meridian

Gall Bladder anger seems to be anger with a target. Usually one of the birth parents is the prototype but it can be more recent people or even a current situation. For example an unmarried pregnant woman whose weakest meridian was GB was very angry with her birth father from events in her childhood; and, currently with the father of her unborn baby who deserted her.

The GB meridian does not respond well to gentle, supportive approaches. The anger or resignation [unhealthy and negative distinction and polarities] must be addressed [in language the GB can understand; that is] sometimes very forcefully.

A seven year old boy with a previously weak Triple Warmer Meridian, showed primary weakness from the GB Meridian after a trip to see his father who was divorced from his mother and living apart. The father had a new wife and he drank much of the time during his son's visit. The boy did not want to talk about the event but after a few minutes of sparring with foam rubber encounter bats [batakas], he no longer showed any Psychological Reversal or a weakened meridian.

A more confrontive and assertive approach is more effective until the meridian's excessive or depleted energy is balanced. Then the client is more open to discussing the conflicting issues disrupting the meridian. This is when the therapist's more nurturing sensitive approach again become useful With PsychoKinesiological techniques these two approaches are integrated... (slightly adapted and reorganized for clarity from p. 142)

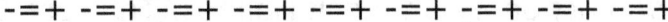

-=+ -=+ -=+ -=+ -=+ -=+ -=+ -=+ -=+

A few words on the Air-Metal element metaphor

It's common to hear in person and see in print very experienced acupuncture practitioners refer to the Air/Metal element. Further complicating the metaphor for persons new to this, the "element" of light, as in "light ether" may be the origin of both the air and metal metaphors. This brings us to air-metal-ether, which you may find useful.

Let's switch to the question of how the lung and large intestine got connected with the Air-Metal element. What if 5,000 years ago, when TCM was developed, what we now call "thinking" was very different than what we call "thinking" today? What if thinking was much more body-centered and connected with these organs? Later thinking "migrated" more fully up into the cerebral nervous system and out of the enteric nervous system.

The modern dilemma is typically human wakefullness has moved too far out of and away from our gut brain. Many males especially have lost awareness of their gut brain intelligences.

"The Enlightenment" of the 1700s pointed to evolving cerebral brain thinking. The full flowering of 'head thinking occurred in old-style physical material science of the 1800s exemplified in fiction by Sherlock Holmes. The "pre-Sherlock Holmes thinking" of TCM still characterizing our lungs & large intestine must therefore be deeply unconscious habits--and so it is.

Dysfunctional axis of the air-metal element ~ Undercharge dysfunction is too loose a hold on your own lessons learned, allowing valuable gem life lessons to slip thru your fingers. Undercharge is too much releasing, too much letting go, not accumulating adequately and sufficiently. Overcharge dysfunction is too tight a hold on values held and life lessons acquired, overly rigid adherence to laws and rules of any kind. Related but different again, the home clutterer, rat-pack pattern: can't let go, can't discern what is waste, what is lessons not yet learned.

The above under- and overcharge expressions can occur on any of three depths, conscious, sub- and unconscious. These dysfunctional patterns can also be written large in local and mainstream cultures.

-=+ -=+ -=+ -=+ -=+ -=+ -=+ -=+

LUNG Meridian & Organ

Air-Metal Yin

Anterior Serratus ~ Coracobrachialis ~ Deltoids ~ Diaphragm

Healthy, positive, balanced is discernment, healthy moral sense, honesty. Mental flexibility. Mental humility, enuf of it to admit, "I don't know, I don't have the information just now." Intellect at its best. Mentally permeable.

Negative emotions absorbed: false pride, disdain, lack of humility; therefore: intolerance, prejudice, contempt, smothered, scorn.

Axis of Dysfunction ~ Habitual sadness and suppressed grief; on the other hand, pride, arrogance, bossy, rigid Law & Order mentality

Other unhealthy expressions: Unconsciously disconnected (from self, from own feelings). Bound by rules no longer cared about nor understood.

Numb UNDER-charged Lung expressions: Loss of zest for life, dispirited. Melancholic thoughts, feels intellectually powerless, intellectually spineless and helpless. May become the victim of abuse of all kinds. Uncommunicative, sullen. Self-expression feels trapped, stifled. Perplexed, emotionally unfulfilled, despair, longing, unhealed separation, not belonging. Feels unappreciated, short-changed by others, feels intellectually insignificant. Unconsciously disappointed. Chronic grief, especially unconscious. Unexpressed mental pain. Compulsive (see also Large Int.)

UNDER-charge Lung coupled with negativity: Disdain, prejudice, contempt.

Numbing OVERcharged Lung expressions: Pride. Proud intellectual arrogance. Rigidly inflexible and single-minded, obstinate and therefore alienated. Senseless heroism. Dogmatic & controlling (see also Large Int).

OVERcharged Lung coupled with negativity: Over-critical. Punishing, vengeful. Uses authority as a weapon (authoritarian). Uses hierarchy as a weapon (hierarchical).

Tales of the Kingdom of Camelot become therapeutic metaphors when we allow Camelot to represent the soul. Merlin's actions illustrate both over- and undercharged air-metal expressions. Whisenant's original insight is King Arthur expresses the air and metal elements. Ten years of clinical experience later, it's clear Merlin is the air-metal element; Arthur is allied with the water element (frozen, fluid or steaming hot). *Whisenant's* insights on Arthur from p. 173 et seq, are transposed to Merlin and expanded on here.

The "Air" element suggests our expansive intellect. When the intellect expresses its soaring, expansive qualities, we have an air expression.

Intellect also has capacity for fierce intention. When the intellect expresses its capacity for fierce intention, we have a sword expression; also, some times a scalpel expression.

Merlin is architect of the future, the architect of Camelot, envisioning it, planning it, tweaking real lives since before Arthur was born. In his intellect he envisions the positive change in the whole of Camelot when all has matured.

Camelot is built upon laws (air), rules (metal) standards and justice instituted by Merlin's wisdom, thru Arthur, to replace "Force Majeur," the more primitive rule of brute force, "might makes right" which preceded the "rule of law" in England. With collective consensus behind it, a rule of laws becomes mightier than any individual with a sword. Wise Socrates died for the sake of group consensus on laws to rule mankind's unbridled passions. Camelot attempts to be the first community ruled by laws, in the West, since the Fall of Rome. Camelot is built by the sword; and then, by the pen.

As he ages, Merlin expresses mostly phases of lung under-charge and becomes weak-willed. He retreats more and more from public life.

When Merlin is stuck

Merlin can be stuck in either over- or undercharge. He doesn't know which direction to go, this way or that way? He feels trapped in his own view of things. He's unable to do reality field testing to clarify what is actually now present.

+ Each heavy metal contains a therapeutic metaphor. For example, the psychology of Zirconium, as in zirconium diamonds, is pride and arrogance.

-=+ -=+ -=+ -=+ -=+ -=+ -=+ -=+ -=+

LARGE INTESTINE Meridian & Organ

Metal-Air Yang

Fascia Lata ~ Hamstrings ~ Quadratus Lumborum

Healthy, positive, balanced: Discriminating is worth holding onto and what must jettisoned as used up. Let go of habits not working for us; and, hold onto habits currently workable for us. Knowing how long to hold on, knowing when to let go.

Mentally permeable. "Humility" captures some of this but 'healthy discrimination' or 'mentally permeable' are closer.

Axis of Dysfunction ~ not holding on to beneficial things long enuf; on the other hand, holding onto things too long.

UNDER- pole dysfunction (1): false sense of powerlessness.

OVER- pole dysfunction (1): false sense of importance

UNDER- pole dysfunction (2): Letting go of mental, emotional, life situations too soon, unable to hold on and to persevere towards personal goals.

OVER- pole dysfunction (2): holds on too long in personal life situations, holds on past and beyond any usefulness, retains useless goods past their expiration date.

Negative emotions absorbed: unconscious holding onto: guilt, regrets, toxic shame, powerlessness.

Other emblematic dysfunction: toxic conditions in the sub- and unconscious.

Neutral UNDERcharged Lg.Int. expressions: Feeling persecuted. Disillusionment leading to withdrawal. Self-imposed isolation. Emotional incontinence (diarrhea). Lack of self-care. Given up, what's the use. "Lowly worm." Feel intellectually impotent. Can be intellectually submissive. Can be the loyal disciple.

Fearing things will be taken away; fears things and people will go away and let's go of them too soon, too detached.

Does not invest them self enuf in relationships, none develop to any depth. Difficulty committing to relationships and to a career. Lacks initiative and openness.

In family of origin: someone bossed them around and possibly TOSSED them around, criticizing all their thoughts and opinions. There was no relaxed, open exchange of ideas, a severe breakdown in exchange of ideas in the family of origin.

UNDER- Lg. Int. metaphors & MYTH: Theseus was not the totally admirable hero commercial versions of the myths portray him as. After Ariadne helps Theseus escape the Labyrinth, he abandons her on an island. Although he promised to marry her, he cannot commit to the relationship. His lack of healthy discrimination is evident in his choice to join the seven Athenian youths selected to be sacrificed to the Minotaur (*Whisenant* 191-194).

Neutral OVERcharge expressions: Over-controlled. Feels coerced or forced. Is dogmatically positioned, unconsciously defended. Arrogance and aloofness (likely compensating for low self-esteem). Difficult to get them into therapy; they try to prove it invalid and useless.

Hoarding & attachment, fearing things will be taken away. Unconscious holding on, uptight, clutching, clinging. Holds onto the current life situation too long, embraces things long past time of diminishing returns. Holds onto dysfunctional relationships. Allows toxic interactions to pile up without any release. Iron-clad. Fear of loss of control. Dominates conversations.

Unconsciously self-righteous, narrow minded, and pedantic. Time urgency. Unmerciful in the sense of unyielding, perfection expectations on self and others. Unconsciously critical.

OVERcharge Lg. Int. expressions coupled with negativity: Tries to control others (uses control as a weapon). Cynical. Defends their being a pack-rat. Expresses disdain. Openly expresses suspicion, scorn, contempt, intolerance and prejudice.

OVERcharged MYTH for Large Intestine: King Minos the tyrant monster, the hoarder of the public good, his ego is a curse to himself and to others. He allows the monster the Minotaur to be created, then does not have the wit to have it destroyed. Thru lack of discrimination he allows his toxic, deadly creation to roam unfettered in the labyrinth (intestines) underground (*Whisenant* 189-191).

Another aspect of King Minos usefully characterizes a common LI overcharge: the ultra-conservative uncritically preserving the status quo, the old-familiar ways in the face of calls for change. Highly assertive, he/she over-controls as many factors as possible to preserve old comfort zones the way they were. Dictator.

+ Brief protocol to assess LI disturbance: make a pie chart of possibly disturbing factors; test for which factor is the "biggest fish". Consider testing for these factors: meridian energetic imbalance, organic physical organ disturbance, Inner

Court fractals in the head, lack of probiotics appropriate for your blood type, other (hidden-cloaked-disguised).

-=+ -=+ -=+ -=+ -=+ -=+ -=+ -=+ -=+

STOMACH Meridian & Organ

Earth Yang

Pectoralis Major Clavicular ~ Levator Scapulae ~ Neck Muscles ~ Brachioradials

Healthy & positive: Pleased, contented, contentment is here or on the way imminently. Perceived proximity of internal needs and external sources of nourishment. Good things are coming to me--like a dog patiently waiting expectantly for a treat.

Satiated, food satisfies. Feeling satisfied here in a 3D human body and human experience. Physical body contentment and tranquility.

Emotions ~ Sensitive to emotional disturbance in self and others. Sympathy-liking, liking and disliking. Deep compassion is not Stomach; it's more Heart.

Taste is a rich metaphor for Stomach dysfunction. As with all meridians, dysfunction is on one side or the other of of too little or too much; either under- or overcharged.

Taste on two levels ~ (1) Healthy taste for things which satisfy the gut-brain, healthy taste for body nourishment, lifestyle and creature comforts. (2) Head-brain: Healthy taste for living, learning, growing serving, healing.

Emblematic dysfunctions: Overcharge: disgusted. Over-sensitive, emotional bleeding, wear your heart on your sleeve, "bleeding heart" (yes, this is really stomach not heart). Undercharge: Starving on multiple levels (starved for touch and affection). Feeling my life cannot be relied upon to meet my needs.

Dysfunction has three phases ~ (1) Too **little** care, concern and TASTE for the emotional needs of your inner child (lack of self-connection). (2) Too much TASTE for the emotional needs of others (over-empathizing, weak interpersonal boundaries, their needs more imprtant than mine). (3) **Too much care**, concern and TASTE for the emotional needs of your child within (caught, stuck, trapped in only first person point of view, only my needs matter).

In the Church of the Perfect Martyr, martyrs perceive other people's lives and other people's problems as tastier than their own issues and their own needs.

Inner Game of Stomach balance is healthy sympathy for our own needs on all levels PACME+Soul.

Outer Game of Stomach balance is healthy sensitivity to the needs of others.

UNDER-charged Stomach dysfunctions

1) Needy, emotional hunger, deprived, neglected, child within feels emotionally empty. Discontented, hidden hungers vaguely driving us.

2) Undernourished, starving, too little taste for body nourishment and healthy creature comforts, achieving internal homeostasis seems hopeless. Self-denial, martyr. Alternatively: Loss of physical appetite, unhealthy weight loss, inability to gain weight. Unable to digest circumstances or situations (unable to process, match feelings with thoughts).

Classic self-denial aspects of the Jewish mother stereotype.

3) Sour on life, sour on relationships. Life and other people leave a bad taste in the mouth. Too little taste for the creature comforts of other people: "Let them eat cake!" Ignoring the basic legitimate hungers of others.

4) Poor social skills. Overly self-absorbed, can only stand-tolerate, the taste of one's own self, dislikes the cooking of other's, eats narrowly. Loss of appetite for 3D life. Gnawing anxiety. Self-neglect.

5) "Too much," overwhelmed, stressed out. Obsesses on one kind of taste too narrowly, taste for only one thing, fanatical (I only desire God; or, Marilyn Monroe, or videogames, or Wall Street success, exaggerated interest in their "hobby horse," too little interest in maturing-up on all levels.

OVER-charged Stomach dysfunctions

Short version ~ Too much awareness of and taste for own creature comforts and/or needs of others. Too much awareness of and taste for the inner (emotional state) of others. Too much awareness of and taste for, resolving outer drama and disturbances in interpersonal situations.

Over-sensitivity to pleasing others, providing for the creature comforts of others, too little attention to pleasing our own child within. Maintaining other people's comfort zones takes up all of our time.

Long version ~

1) Mild obsession; as in, men chasing women; and, men chasing women's breasts. The chase and the honeymoon as peak experience men shoot for (taste for the hunt). Hyped up, overcharged stomach energy petering out. After the honeymoon, marriage begins, peak romance ends and men can lose interest "the thrill is gone."

2) Over-liking unhealthy foods, over-liking unhealthy relationships, liking what is not good for us. Related to enabling behaviors. Active disgust with our lot in life (also check spleen and gall bladder on this).

2) Active-heightened over-sensitivity to family, friends and colleagues. Too much taste for things in the Outer Game of Life. This often compensates for too little attention paid to the Inner Game of Life.

Nosy, intrusive, overly-attached-to-others aspects of the Jewish mother stereotype. See also overcharged thyroid: "all about me," the Drama Queen," who needs to monopolize all attention in a room of people.

3) Active over-sensitivity and over-caring for the poor, the downtrodden, victims, homeless and stray animals, of all sizes. This can become an obsession. If so check if the person is doing on the outside, externally, what needs to be done on the inside, internally.

4) Obsessing to get a specific need-hunger met. Commonly seen in the male stereotype of chasing (hungering for) women who satisfy a hidden HUNGER for a warm, nurturing mother the man never had. Hence the obsession with big breasts in the U.S. Similarly, the obsession with sex-with-another as an image-metaphor for the deeper hidden hunger for intimacy and connecting with our own child within. The fascination, potential obsession, of older men with younger women, who represent and express own lost physical-etheric vitality.

"Co-dependency" is a useful term but not precise enuf for disturbances of Stomach, Pancreas and Spleen.

UNDERcharged dysfunction coupled with spleen overcharge negativity: Smoldering hatred

UNDER- metaphors and MYTHS for Stomach: The Hypochondriac, overly attentive to personal deficit. Feeling deprived, empty, hungry for contact and nourishment. Whining or demanding to be filled up by others, Jewish American Princess stereotype. Out of touch with the needs of others.

The martyr, taste for self-sacrifice, self-sacrifice made into a virtue, for any reason. Whisenant's representation of Jesus here is deliberately one-sided, only the martyr is considered, Jesus as "The meek shall inherit the Earth," the "turn the other cheek" Jesus, the continually self-sacrificing one. The Jesus of the Matthew

Testament, the Sacrificial Lamb, helping others with little concern for self. Turn the other cheek, "Do not resist evil." When you get crucified, smile.

In the Church of the Perfect Martyr, the martyr perceives other people's lives and other people's problems, as tastier than their own issues and their own needs. Expressions of excessive self-sacrifice are sometimes on display in victims of wife-beating and enablers of dysfunction in others: Over-attention to other's needs + self-neglect. The Jewish Mother stereotype who "dies" over and over again in service to her son, other people, etc. (adapted from *Whisenant* 211).

A martyr arranges things so someone else gets their needs met, not the martyr. A martyr does not have themselves in their own picture of contentment and success. Their pictures of happiness and success are only *other* people happy and successful.

Whisenant mentions Karen Carpenter and her Anorexia Nervosa: Loss of appetite, no taste for food, legs seem weak. weight loss. Karen Carpenter was likely out on both spleen and stomach. Overly attendant to needs of others, over-generous and neglectful of self.

Other OVERcharged Stomach behavior: Similar to spleen, too much attention is projected outward: over-concern with needs of others, too little caution for self, too little care of self.

OVERcharge Stomach coupled with negativity: Active disgust, active revulsion. Excess antipathy: "Yuck!" Active loathing, including self-loathing. Toxic-acid hatred, "she has an acid tongue" (compare with Gall Bladder's "smart bomb anger"). The parts of us handling stomach acid appear to absorb toxic disgust & revulsion. Some over-acid stomachs are expressing toxic judgment, bitterness, gut revulsion, of self, others, the world, or God.

Other disturbed Stomach emotions absorbed, difficult to categorize by the above: fickle and nausea.

OVER- Stomach metaphors & MYTHS: Romans at the time of Christ, greedy, self-serving stance of some Jews and Romans at the time of Christ.

+ In highly overcharged state, stomach meridians can be outside the physical body, in front, and flowing up instead of peacefully down. Meridian tracing, visualization; plus, saying, "God bless me, I love me, peace is present" can help.

+ Most sensitive to emotional disturbance, in self and others, of all meridians. Stomach meridian is the meridian of the Inner Child to an astonishing degree. When tears exit the eye at the middle bottom, they trace exactly the beginning of the stomach meridian. This can also be seen in some mime face painting of tears.

Like overcharged Spleen-Pancreas, overcharged STOMACH projects awareness outward: over-concern with needs of others, too little care, taste, comfort, caution for self.

+ Absence of stomach in TCM: Herbalist Matthew Wood observes how TCM, developed 5000 to 2000 years ago, virtually ignores the stomach organ and stomach meridian function. The stomach is deeply personal. Traditional ancient Chinese culture (Confucius) is deeply impersonal. Since the "Me generation," it's very relevant to expand our understanding of Stomach Meridian psychology.

+ Stomach meridian running backwards as "too many big ideas." A large-scale polarity imbalance can exist this way: on one side difficulty taking in physical nourishment, underweight, low physical vitality; on the other side, voracious appetite for BIG ideas in a certain area of interest. This can be computers, as in the classic skinny nerd; but can also be, fantasy & science fiction as in the classic sci-fi nerd (please excuse any seeming judgment. This is me also, a recovering New Age/spirituality nerd).

+ The fun part here is looking for where a person has a taste for "big ideas" compensating for lack of physical nourishment and self-care.

+ Whisenant mentions Schizophrenia as at the far end of stomach imbalance. The present author is more aligned with Mimi Castellanos and NLP. Mimi points to the bladder meridian as more at cause in Schizophrenia, a water element problem. NLP points to sub-modality strategies to dissociate from the physical body.

-=+ -=+ -=+ -=+ -=+ -=+ -=+ -=+ -=+

SPLEEN-PANCREAS Meridian & Organs

Earth Yin

Latisimus Dorsi ~ Middle Trapezius ~ Lower Trapezius

~ Opponens Polliccis Longus ~ Triceps

Healthy headline (positive & balanced): Contentment. Perceived goodness. Healthy attention to self, healthy self-care. Outwardly, appropriate sympathy and nurturing of others. Singing: "Full of the sweet nectar of life. "My Girl:" 'I've got so much honey, the bees envy me'" (*Whisenant* p. 220). Faith and confidence in one's future, self-assurance.

Note: "the milk of human kindness" is not spleen but is right and left pericardium meridians.

Negative headline ~ Hiding your light under a bushel, especially emotionally, hiding how you feel from others. *Therefore* depressed. Guilting yourself for your troubles whether justified or not.

More positives

Harmonious, peace-maker, resonates well with others. Awake and aware to your own needs and to the needs of other's. Ability to resonate with others and arrange for them to resonate with you.

Accepting, open feelings, harmony, appropriate consideration of others. Interest in and dedication to others. Healthy role-playing, creates beneficial roles in life useful and beneficial to self, family and others; therefore, faith and confidence in one's future.

Healthy, safe, trustworthy, contented togetherness: "I like you. Let's be friends. Let's hold hands." Many children, especially around age five, do this with other children near their own age; they are able to "resonate together." Happy children's songs.

+ Muscle metaphor for LATISSIMUS DORSI- This muscle extends from the back from the hip to the spine and to the shoulder and is involved in all the movements of the arm across the front of the body. When it is out of balance posture is effected from the shoulders to the pelvis. Feel this muscle contracting at the side of the back when the elbow is held tightly against the body, arm straight, with the thumb pointing to the back.

[Overcharge:] Trying to embrace too much, are you taking swings at life which are too big, overblown? Are you blaming others for what you dislike in your life? In "The Taming of the Shrew," the angry throwing of dishes, striking out at others, instead of reflective consideration of your part in creating what life brings to you.

[Balance:] Embracing all of my life appropriately.

[Undercharge:] Needing to open my arms wider to embrace more of my life, are you inhibited from making large gestures towards reaching your goals?

(Above adapted from Matthew Thie *T4H* 2nd Ed p 125; and, T4H newsletter, 1999).

Headline disturbed Overcharged expression: Women throwing dishes. This is projecting blame. Also check Liver for rage. Trump made blame fashionable again; long-term, it is immature and can only become destructive.

Therapists and healers often learn angry feelings (liver-gallbladder) held in the sub- and unconscious, do not track back to present events. The anger is often unresolved from the client's past, often distant past.

Blame (spleen) can be the same way, its origin in past unresolved hurts. If you subject yourself to intense emotional pressures, taking too much personal responsibility (feeling guilty) for what life brings you, this dampens your healthy spleen energy of contentment.

Therapists servicing clients with suicidal ideation commonly uncover repressed rage (live-gallbladder) and repressed blame (spleen) from long ago incidents.

Our feminine (*yin*) destructive and self-destructive expressions are culturally unpopular. They are dismissed and repressed. Self-loathing energy can be "banished," pushed down in the body, towards the calves, ankles, feet.

"Blowing off steam" can be release of either no longer necessary spleen or liver-gallbladder disturbances. Check to see if the disturbance releasing is right or left-sided before you decide which organ is disturbed.

Negative psychology absorbed: anxiety, for pancreas especially: feeling my life is out of my control; others are in control of me. When spleen meridian runs backwards and is overcharged, we have High Anxiety; as if, standing on top of a 12 foot A-frame ladder, where it's unsafe, with nothing at all to hold onto for support, madly looking for where stability lies.

Axis of dysfunction: under pole: withdrawing into my inner world, withholding from self, ultimately withholding from myself the Sun's prana of ripeness, roundness and fullness.

Over pole: over-giving to the needs of others (See also Stomach and too much taste for the concerns of others).

UNDER- pole Spleen dysfunction (1): Trouble saying "yes"

OVER- pole Spleen dysfunction (1): trouble saying "no."

UNDER- pole Spleen dysfunction (2): Retreating into a cave of introversion, living there; consequently, under-caring for self and/or others

OVER- pole Spleen dysfunction (2): Over-caring for self or others. Note how these two together contribute to the Jewish Mother stereotype.

UNDER- pole Spleen dysfunction (3): Deficient role-playing in life reducing getting your own needs met.

OVER- pole Spleen dysfunction (3): Excessive role-playing reducing getting your own needs met.

UNDER- pole Spleen dysfunction (4): feels smothered

OVER- pole Spleen dysfunction (4): smothering behavior.

Other UNDERcharged behavior: Poor or negative self-image: Other people see me as unattractive, as a failure, etc. and I'm stuck with how they see me, stuck with living in people's low opinion of me. Pensiveness, taking public disapproval "to heart," feel incapable of re-inventing their image and how they come across to others.

The pancreas in undercharge feels out of control, feels other people are in control of me, others are in control of my life, not me (Mimi Castellanos). Trouble saying "Yes," over-concern with details, restless with unconscious anxiety; therefore, always dissatisfied. Tendency to hold things inside, inability to blow off steam (as in vent one's spleen by throwing dishes).

Over-concern and worry about others, attempts to control things which cannot be controlled, classically one's own grown-up children.

Tendency to eat quickly, while doing other things; overeats because not paying enuf attention to self and body. Overuse of the mind and under-use of body; won't exercise. Difficulty reaching out to new sources of life enhancement, never feeling full. Fear destruction and don't know why (may point to early childhood and prior existences).

Collapsed personal boundaries. Feel inadequate, not good enuf, feel empty, feel deprived, low self-esteem. Out of touch with needs of self and others. Boundary issues. Difficulty starting and/or bringing relationships to an end.

A woman's experience of living in a man's world. Feeling lost in a harsh male world, lost in a world not of my own making or values.

The Satir Stress-Response-Stance of the Placator.

Hypochondriac. May whine, preoccupied with dysfunction, what's not working, Feel run down even if not, nerves are going to pieces. Does not chew and digest things sufficiently. Lacks perseverance to fully assimilate things. Excessive worry. Too dependent on others, does not trust themself and own ability. Interferes with work of others.

Martyr. Living thru other people's happiness and success.

Co-dependence. Dependent, clingy. Emotionally anxious, distressed feelings, unfounded fears. Self-delusion corrupts playing beneficial role in relationship. Enabling disabilities in their spouse. May believe "I must take care of them or they will leave me." Doormat, feel they deserve abuse. Loss of healthy self-image.

Enablers, may believe "I must take care of them or they will leave me."

Healers who need to heal themselves more, overly attendant to the needs of others, over-generous, lacking healthy unconscious boundaries. Healers who give until they burn out.

Bruce speculates most professional counselors and intuitive healers start out as co-dependent. They have to learn alertness to fuzzy boundaries and self-denial this lifetime. See also the topic of iNtuitive Feelers, "NFs" in MBTI; and, Highly Sensitive Persons in Judith Orloff.

Wallflower. Tendency not to talk to others and remain alone. Fear, as in trouble saying "Yes." Hesitant, timid, overly careful and cautious

Hermit. Recluse, tend to avoid people, more contented alone. "I vant to left alone!" ~ Greta Garbo. Awareness of your own unresolved, toxic internal parts, unwillingness to expose these with others. "Stay away from me!" Overly self-absorbed.

Homeless derelicts. "Life is pointless, too silly to care about at all." Neglects playing any beneficial role whatsoever. Emotionally devastated. Possible clinical depression.

UNDERcharge Spleen myths: Orpheus and the music of the spheres. Orpheus is the harmonizer but one-sided in his capacity. He provides the healthy resonance and knitting together the crew of the Argo needs to face dangers. However Orpheus lacks the leadership qualities of Jason, who represents right side and liver. Orpheus' excesses are passive excesses, lack of strong personal boundaries and lack of strong, healthy heterosexual polarity (*Whisenant* 225 et seq).

+ Diabetes ~ Broken power & broken dreams; i.e., "I can't have my own dreams." Chronic dis-contentment, dis-empowerment, disappointment. "I don't get to do what I wanted to do in life." These are prime common factors in diabetic psychology.

Advertising co-opts our unique dreams, replacing them with standardized dreams: dream of having THIS; dream THIS WAY.

We crave sweet foods to compensate for the lost sweetness of life. Life is only sweet when we acknowledge our dream, put action on it, and follow0-thru with consistent baby-steps. It's a cinch by the inch.

From Medical Intuitive Lynne Boutross, diabetes as not wanting to grow up emotionally, stuck in teenage emotionality [and dissatisfaction]. Not feeling comfortable with surroundings [going sour on self or surroundings].

+ Serotonin appears to be the neurotransmitter most connected with the spleen meridian. Check for EXCESS serotonin in gut.

+ Spleen as receiver of solar prana ~ The spleen etheric center is where the Sun's etheric forces are stepped down and enter the human etheric body to be distributed.

Clairvoyants tell us the physical spleen organ is the physical level of our energetic opening and connection with the Sun's etheric vitality. Consider a peach. How does it ripen and become round? It takes in the Sun's ripening and roundness. The spleen is the most receptive and sensitive to invisible etheric energy, closest to the cosmic, closest to receiving prana, closest of the lower organs to being cosmic.

This clarifies the TCM idea of spleen as healthy roundness—not obesity or plumpness. The elderly or anyone with compromised intake of etheric vitality thru the spleen portal, affect a thinner, angular physical bearing.

+ Like earthly plants who's only possible response to life and circumstances is to grow, the Spleen only response can be love. It only knows how to give. This is why trouble saying "no," and trouble saying "yes" are spleen issues more than heart issues. The loving nature of the heart appears to be at an altogether more conscious level. Spleen giving or withholding is more sub- and unconscious.

+ Stephen Lewis in *Sanctuary* says in diabetes cases, check for TB in pancreas. he says this relates to sugar addiction. If left unchecked, it can progress to diabetes.

+ In early childhood and/or prior existences felt food; and/or, social & emotional nourishment, could not be trusted, was invalid somehow. Gave up on reaching out.

+ Overlap with Stomach Meridian issues: Bruce suggests omentum, stomach, pancreas and spleen are the four organs representing receptive capacity to feeling in the body. These organs "progress" from most alert and awake (omentum) to most unconscious, ancient and asleep (spleen).

The omentum is a flap of nerve tissue overhanging the stomach in front. This is the main quantity of nerve tissue comprising the enteric nervous system (ENS) or "gut brain." This is where we feel butterflies in the stomach and hit in the gut, not the stomach so much. The omentum is closest to the front surface and is the most conscious of our organs charged with receptivity; keeping in mind, the most conscious of these organs remains SUBconscious.

Stomach is the next deepest organ. It's response is difficult to distinguish from the omentum as the omentum covers the stomach and has much more nerve tissue then the stomach per se. Older literature lumps stomach and omentum together and with some justification.

Pancreas is the next deepest organ of receptivity. It's issues are difficult to distinguish from the spleen; both of them relate to the Earth qualities of emotional "warmth" and "sweetness" in the psyche.

+ Persons whose health issues are primarily left-sided

Many people have decidedly more right or more left-sided health issues. A left-sided "preference" for health issues suggests weakness in Guinevere and Merlin in the Inner Court of the gut brain. See the Inner Court book for more.

+ Spleen & liver as emotional filters

Above the belly button and below the heart, in the enteric nervous system, the spleen and liver filter unresolved emotions circulating in the energetic body.

+ Spleen as ancient emotion

In ancient times, earlier phases of human evolution, the spleen was apparently the seat of our early emotional life. What we know today as "heart feelings" were earlier, only in our spleen. Our awareness of our feelings was lower in our body, in the spleen.

Today we feel our deep emotions higher in our bodies, at the level of the heart and lungs. This explains the curious avoidance in TCM of stomach emotions, the more personalized form of feelings (me, me, me) we are more familiar with today. It may be human emotional awareness over ages moved towards the front of the body and higher in the body.

Spleen was also the filter for unresolved emotions. Our spleen today remains a repository for ancient unresolved emotions. It's possible to clear deeply unconscious feelings-emotions, stuck in the emotional filter of the spleen.

+ Spleen and hormones ~ Several sources say if you wish to address hormones, address the spleen meridian.

+ Spleen is the the bright, but not too bright, light of the sun. Pancreas is the sweetness of life. Stomach is nourishment and satisfying tastes. These sensations characterize Guinever in the gut brain.

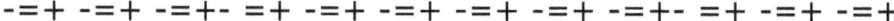

-=+ -=+ -=+- =+ -=+ -=+ -=+ -=+ -=+ -=+- =+ -=+ -=+

A few words on the water element

A full human life will have times to feel both over and undercharge in the water element.

It will have time to feel bladder undercharge: Child-like euphoria, extreme relaxation and lack of worry, "Peel me a grape," Flower child, Flow Child, in love with everything, absence of responsibility to others, the world and career.

It may also have time to feel unhealthy kidney overcharge: you with a 12 foot tall, A-frame ladder, climbing to the top, then climbing higher, beyond safety, to stand on the tippy-top of the ladder, with no handholds anywhere, madly surveying your environment for outer support, in your moment of crisis.

A full life may also have time to feel healthy bladder charge: competence, confidence, courage, healthy arousal in your own professional field, setting and striding forward towards goals, an effective athlete in your profession, with passion for today's baby-step tasks.

The water element expands the simple imagery of under and overcharge used with the other meridians. With water, ALL physical states, solid crystal, flowing liquid, gaseous, has positive and negative expressions in our psyche.

Mimi Castellanos says not wanting to be seen or to be present connect to bladder and kidney meridians dysfunction. Stifling our basic self-support instincts in order to protect ourself was the historical norm of mass consciousness up to the early 1970s. In the early 1970s, "do your own thing" came to life. Self-support and self-expression began to be redeemed. In past times, a peasant appearing before the King, the Lord, the Baron, the appropriate way to feel was less-than, subservient, ashamed, lowly, the necessity to hide both the good and bad of your inner self, so it won't be used against you in the eyes of the powerful and capricious, who have control of your life and livelihood

-=+ -=+ -=+ -=+ -=+ -=+ -=+ -=+ -=+

BLADDER Meridian & Organ

Water Yang

Peroneus ~ Sacrospinalis ~ Tibials

Healthy, positive, balanced expression: Healthy inner cooperation between conscious-waking self above and inner child below; therefore, self trust and courage. The ordinariness of healthy inner cooperation, healthy inner balance, healthy inner tension, healthy caution. The open focus and relaxed enthusiasm of a child *(Whisenant),* especially children in the "golden age of Childhood, age 10-11, just before puberty.

As adults, confidence, balanced between standing up for yourself without imposing yourself on others. Easily moving between fluidity and ice, between spontaneity and solid resolution, as free as the wind and as solid as a rock.

UNDER- pole dysfunction (1): overly fluid

OVER- pole dysfunction (1): ice, overly rigid, inflexible. Trying, especially "trying to be someone" different from who you are.

UNDER- pole dysfunction (2): no tension at all, limp resolution about everything, lowered conscious arousal, "whatever" and, "It can wait, I'll do it tomorrow" about everything. Calm serenity taken to extremes.

OVER- pole dysfunction (2): Cannot relax vigilance, addicted to trying, restless, impatient. Tongue sticking out during times of unconscious concentration, constant intensity, intensity over-applied. See also KO cycle: overthinking of Earth element reduces water element.

Negative emotions absorbed: fear of external things and threats, anxiety; therefore, dread & impatience.

Other UNDERcharged behavior: "I can't," disruption of healthy confidence and courage: vacillation, fearful, frozen willingness, taken aback.

UNDERcharged BL MYTH: Flower Child, Flow Child. Trusting and in love with everything and everyone. Childlike in all ways both desirable and undesirable. Immature discretion. No drive to set and achieve major goals. Ignore responsibility; if I'm not responsible, no urgency at all for anything. See also Down's Syndrome kids. If their needs are not provided by a benefactor, they can only live a meager 3D existence.

Fairy tale: "The Boy who wanted to learn fear" in *Italian Folktales*, too little caution, oblivious to all and every danger, out of touch with his own feeling of fear and needs for safety (because he lives only in his head, in his thoughts).

Other OVERcharged behavior: Wants to perfect self in image of parent or hero.

OVERcharged BL MYTH: Superheroes as in, "I want to be *somebody*!" Lone Ranger, Batman, Joker, etc., especially in the hero role of "guardian of Gotham or Metropolis." Stiff, stereotyped behavior, follows an image of high self-concept slavishly, cook book fashion, excessive comparison of self to others and to one's own high standards (check imposed unhealthy adult criteria for "goodness" in early family of origin).

Since Bladder Meridian and Governing Vessel are located in same area of body, dysfunctions can be hard to separate.

Bladder meridian overcharge is often accompanied by chronic muscle tension. Pervasive problems of over-stress and back discomfort can develop. Lacks healthy spontaneity, replaces it with merely erratic behavior.

The literature of non-sense

On the Writer's Almanac, Garrison Keillor profiled humorist Will Cuppy. I remembered Cuppy fondly from my youth. His ilk includes the humorist P.G. Wodehouse, who wrote for the Marx brothers, the Marx brothers themselves, and Ogden Nash.

A pattern exists here, a genre of literature was called "light verse." It's possible it's more accurate the genre expresses bladder meridian running backwards, the literature of non-sense. "Jabberwocky."

Cuppy and Nash stand out to me because their verbal patterns are perceptible. Their humor is more often than not, built upon non-sequiturs, deliberately leading in one direction; then, the pay-off makes a left turn, NOT making sense, deliberately breaking sense in favor of non-sense.

"Breaking up sense" is close to "breaking up integrity" and this uncovers the dysfunctional bladder meridian connection. See also, Virginia Satir's Distractor stress response pattern.

FYI Cuppy never married and eventually committed suicide.

The female pattern of dysfunctional bladder meridian may differ significantly. Comments from women invited.

Reading more of Nash, it occurs to me another pattern may be disembodiment, aiming awareness away from and apart from the physical body, dissociating from the 3D physical world.

I recall looking at and reading books by these guys in sixth grade in my all-boy school. In my class, there were 3 or 4 of us who were very taken with nonsense in all its forms. Looking back, we classmates more attracted to nonsense were the ones more in process with flexible thinking, thinking outside the box, a two-edged sword leading to both mental illness--and genius.

Bladder meridians and mental illness

To discuss the role of bladder meridians holistically here, we need a clear definition of the range of mental illness:

Mental Illness disrupts a person's ability to relate to others and function daily. Just as diabetes is a disturbance of blood sugar regulation, mental illnesses results in diminished capacity for coping with the ordinary demands thinking and feeling clearly, being able to match a thought with a feeling; and, a feeling with thoughts. Undesirable behaviors occur when mental-emotional disturbances become habitual.

In *NEW Energy Anatomy*, mental illness is primarily a top~bottom disturbance. Bladder meridians run from head to foot. Think: **dissociation**, dissociating head-brain from gut-brain, CNS from ENS. Dissociation between head and gut is relevant in hyperactivity all the way up to schizophrenia.

Bladder meridians appear to pertain to; and, highly interactive with, the entire range of mental illness.

Mental disturbances from subtle to major are reflected in disturbed bladder meridian flow. Speculation here is, while mental illness can show up in other meridians-organs, it may be, bladder meridians are the main meridians where dissociation (mental illness) shows up. (Notes from Mimi Castellanos of HealthyEnergetics.net were instrumental to the thinking in this paragraph).

Other energetic Bladder lore

+ *Whisenant* observes just about every American patient he sees has over-charged bladder. Bruce observes a large percentage of people in the US trying to unconsciously force this meridian to run UP hill, against its natural flow. This is an immature strategy to grab "more energy." See also Superman-in-action in Governing Vessel section, above.

+ Mimi Castellanos connects bladder and kidney meridian dysfunction with mental illness, schizophrenia and bi-polar tendencies. "I am treating this with a neurotransmitter support from Apex called Acetlechol Tone, neurotransmitter nutrition."

+ Bladder meridian psych ~ "Typically if we have an imbalanced bladder meridian we will be concerned with energy on an almost existential level – wondering if we have the strength to carry on. The nightmare this can turn into for some, is a parched and paranoid terror of fearing for our lives. We can become frantic in seeking the barest scrap of refreshment and energy. Yet an immature bladder meridian function can never hold water actively. Water literally slips through our fingers. Energetically there is a level of trust and surrender required to be able to hold water be a steady container vessel, a grail, to hold the waters of life.

Consider on land, hard, dry earth, deflects sudden rains, no penetration, no holding. For energy NOT to move on by, pass us by, we need a discipline of surrender and permeability. "water" represents our capacity to hold onto [etheric vitality] within our energy field' (Paul Hougham in *The Atlas of Mind, Body and Spirit* p156 edited for clarity by the present author) - https://fiveseasonsmedicine.com/the-bladder-meridian-the-autonomic-nervous-system/

+ UNDERcharged Cycle of Fear and the Bladder

Few things disturb our spiritual well being more than feeling we have little or no energy at any level, accompanied with a sense of internal panic and raciness, and feel unable to meet life on its terms. We may freeze in fear or thrash about in fear, imagining ourselves alone, isolated, beyond help, facing a terrifying future. Everything and everyone seems a threat. We wish to hide, need to rest, long for hibernation, hoping to restore our reserves. We become preoccupied with self-preservation. As our resources diminish still further, our will to live diminishes as well.

OVERcharged Cycle of Fear and the Bladder

Bravado as Opposite Bladder Imbalance:

In the opposite extreme, overcharged Bladder meridian can manifest as a lack of fear. Rather than a grounded, healthy expression of appropriate courage in circumstances, one puts on a mask of disinterest, detachment or active bravado. False bravado is an effort to avoid feeling your own fear.

Fear is healthy when it serves to protect our physical body. Or, fear can be irrational, imagined as lurking in the muddy water, terrifying, just below the waterline. The more unresolved fear in our UNconscious, the more likely we are to display outward fearlessness, act out a tough protective role. This can manifest as the extreme practice of martial arts, body building, collecting guns, ammunition, weapons, being in a violent gang, or engaging in extreme sports and activities such as bungie jumping - https://fiveseasonsmedicine.com/the-bladder-meridian-the-autonomic-nervous-system/

-=+ -=+ -=+ -=+ -=+ -=+ -=+ -=+ -=+

KIDNEY Meridian & Organs

Water, Yin, Flows up from feet

Psoas ~ Upper Trapezius ~ Illacus

Healthy, positive expressions: Self-support, healthy connection to both YANG and *yin*. Therefore, inwardly resourceful, inwardly connected; YANG and *yin* are my friends and I am supported by both. YANG and *yin* flow into me, thru me then into the world. Confidence in how I get my own needs met.

Ability to take healthy personal responsibility for my getting my own needs met, RIGHT and left. Absence of compulsive-obsessive dependence on external support of any kind. Loyalty to my own needs; therefore, possible to understand others have their own needs. Healthy resolution of power disputes.

Willingness to express YANG or *yin* as appropriate in the moment, appropriate responses to 3D living and relationships. Calm and steady when appropriate, wild and engaged when appropriate, without self-excessive consciousness. Absence of arrogance or pushy because can always find a way to flow around obstacles. Engaged appropriately, neither clinging nor aloof. Trust.

Overcharge dysfunction: trusting too much, trusting too long. Undercharge dysfunction: no trust, mistrust, suspicion.

Healthy sexual congress: trusting self, trusting another, letting another in appropriately; hence, healthy boundaries.

Dysfunctional expressions: insecurities, anxiety, internal fears, phobias, mistrust of own habits, unhealthy ambitions, worships graven images, superstitious.

When kidney meridians run backward and are overcharged, this is you, climbing to the top of a 12 foot tall, A-frame ladder; then, climbing higher, beyond safety, to stand on the tippy-top of the ladder, with no handholds anywhere, madly surveying your environment for outer support, in your moment of crisis. This is perceived absence of support from either YANG or *yin* inside.

In moments of crisis, absent internal support, every person and everything is evaluated only in the light of, "Can they help me get my needs met!?" If "no" then in overcharge, it's possible to push them away. If "yes," then in overcharge, you attach to them; the outer attachment compensates for lack of inner self-support.

Other emblematic dysfunctions: Over-caution: Fear of the Boogy Man! Monsters under the bed; fear of the unknown.

Richard Utt on kidney meridian psychology: sexual (in)security, creative, (in)security, (over)caution, careless, (in)decisive, (un)loyal, suspicion.

Axis of dysfunction ~ Note: So far we have figured out only the YANG half of Axis of Dysfunction: On one hand no ambition, no passion, no drive. On the other hand, all about ambition, power, passion and drive, even to a murderous degree.

UNDERcharge YANG connection: aimless, no aspiration at all, no ambition. Actions and efforts are not well planned and executed; does not plan for a positive future. Full of remorse, obsesses on emotional losses. Unresolved deep emotional losses known from this lifetime; or, deeply unconscious, even from prior existences.

OVERcharge YANG connection: high-driving, ruthless, no compromise at all. See right and left sided expressions:

Kidney meridian dysfunction seems to have very decided yang and yin expressions, right and left-sided expressions. Our language for these disturbances is masculine and feminine; still, women can have either; men can have either.

Masculine overcharged kidney expressions

"Ruthless ambition, drive to acquire things and trophies, to the point of "ambition for blood." Ambition to the point of kill-or-be-killed. Grandiose aspirations; wants more of everything. Wants to start at the top in their career and can justify this abundantly. Great expectations of achievement. Can block their own fears by searching for new and different things to conquer." Adamant about what they want and think others stand in their way. Feel others hinder them in life--thus avoiding facing their own fears. Major life accomplishments accompanied by a trail of wreckage in their personal life. Uses everyone around them as pawns in relentless struggle for goals and recognition. Sexual drive and greed for conquest. Potential for brutality, wife beating. The berserker warrior, fighting irrationally (from *Whisenant*, revised and expanded).

The Rolling Stones' "Satisfaction" song is emblematic of disturbed overcharge kidney meridians. "Satisfaction" expresses a good deal of classic kidney meridian imbalance and overcharge.

Kidney overcharge is expressed in the over-frustration over-ambition of the line, "I can't get no satisfaction" and especially in the lines, "I'm tryin' to make some girl, who tells me, 'Baby, better come back, maybe next week,' Can't you see I'm on a losing streak?" Deep satisfaction eludes and escapes me because I'm all YANG and without any nourishing *yin*.

Feminine overcharged kidney expressions

Self-loathing. "I hate myself; I hate my life," dwell on how dissatisfied they are with the present life situation. *Fear and Loathing in Las Vegas* expresses this frequency. Very active mistrust, possibly to the point of paranoia. Related to women throwing dishes to vent.

UNDERcharged kidney behavior (for both *yin* and YANG): Lack of acceptance of adult status: fear of commitment. Classic underachievers, feels inadequate and inferior. Little motivation to try again at goals. 'Incapable of taking action,' incapable of standing up for self. Timid and shy. Relationships feel like foreign territory. Chronic and repressed disappointment. Withholding all feelings. Hiding emotional wounds.

Overworks, exhausts self. Efforts poorly planned and executed. Loss of determination and drive. Lacks courage, self-confidence, sexual interest. Guilt. "Allergic" to bad news.

UNDERcharge KIDNEY MYTH from Whisenant: House of Atreus. Orestes is sent away from the House of Atreus as a child. He only returns when his father is murdered by his mother. He is aimless, has no aspiration at all for himself, no ambition. He is confronted with the task of avenging his father's murder at the cost of murdering his mother. He is obsessed with guilt and remorse and can generate no direction in his life (*Whisenant* 289-292).

OVERcharge KIDNEY MYTH (1): Tantalus was a son of Zeus. He was the only mortal allowed to eat with the gods at their table. Sometimes they came to eat at his table. Believe it or not, in the story Tantalus kills his only son, Pelops, boils him and serves him to the gods at a dinner party. His motivation is unclear. Whisenant connects this extreme behavior with the ruthlessness, jealousy, hatred, audacity, foolhardiness and arrogance of overcharged [yang] kidney meridian (289-291).

Overcharge KIDNEY MYTH (2): Whisenant also mentions the book, *Mommie Dearest* (1984), the harrowing portrait by the daughter of Joan Crawford: "A parent can become so engrossed in attaining goals and recognition, children are used as pawns in the parent's relentless struggle to climb the social ladder" (*Whisenant* 286).

Other energetic Kidney lore

+ TCM believes kidney meridian is the first meridian formed in utero. If true, this would make it the expression of our very most unconscious habit patterns.

+ Kidney meridian travels approximately the full length of the psoas muscles on either side, perhaps the deepest muscles in the human body.

+ The psoas connect emotionally, with the two poles of fear (Right side:)

fear of being engulfed, eaten up, obliterated, absorbed by a more powerful being, one's own identify absorbed into another more powerful identity not your own. (Left side:) fear of total abandonment, being totally alone, forgotten, bereft, life limited to only the resources and perspective of your own limited, small "s" identity.

+ Kidneys are bi-lateral, a pair, a team. Where do they learn to work as a team? From the relationship of your birth mother and father in the first two years. Was your parents' relationship stressed at that time, dysfunctional, conflicted? This will tend to be absorbed and then played back by the kidneys.

One way to check this is to test and see if the two kidneys know about each other. One often is hyper, working overtime, the other kidney is hypo, looking elsewhere. Either or both kidney may be unaware it has a partner, a teammate.

+ Our deeper unconscious kidney issues are in part formed and "programmed in" during our nine months of pregnancy and in the first hour after the first breath. This is when a large fraction of our unconscious habits re-establish themselves.

+ We "sponge up" unconscious habit patterns from both our birth mother and birth father.

+ Merlin represents the left kidney in the Inner Court. This is consistent with all TCM concepts of kidney yin. King Arthur represents the right kidney in the Inner Court, consistent with all TCM concepts of kidney yang.

+ Left kidney can be unconscious fear of being wrong; or, fear of not being right. One manifestation of this is Merlin as dysfunctional preacher, unwittingly teaching out of negativity, unaware the ideas he espouses track back to negativity and to downward spirals.

+ Right kidney can be righteousness; as in, "I know I'm right, just because I know I'm right," negative conviction, unsupported self-conviction. The more familiar expression of this is in overcharge.

+ Righteousness on the right can cover up and compensate for feeling wrong and undeserving felt on the left side. These two together suggest the classic dysfunctional preacher pattern.

+ Right kidney is also SELF DOUBT, a psychological plague assigned to Arthur in Arthurian legend.

+ Mimi Castellanos connects bladder and kidney meridian dysfunction with mental illness and bi-polar tendencies. She reports, "I am treating this with a neurotransmitter support from Apex called Acetlechol Tone, I think, part of their neurotransmitter nutrition. I love Apex products."

+ More on "kidney undercharge:" Both YANG and *yin can be* undercharged at deeply unconscious level represented in the kidneys. When disturbances are this unconscious, both ends of the see saw appear Externally. One end of the seesaw, kidney undercharge can appear as "stick in the mud" unwillingness to change. On the other end of the seesaw, is attraction to elves and fairies: ElfQuest, Lord of the Rings elves, elves in DragonAge videogames. Note the thin arms and general lack of physical development of elves, undernourished energetically.

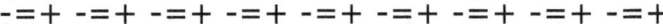

-=+ -=+ -=+ -=+ -=+ -=+ -=+ -=+ -=+

Balancing disturbed meridians

Many methods now exist to balance disturbed meridians. One is acupuncture. This can work and your insurance may pay for it. Some people needle themselves. More people use these methods:

- Meridian tracing ala Donna Eden at http://www.innersource.net/innersource more simple than...

- Neuroenergetic Kinesiology

- Other methods of Meridian Tracing; including, guided creative visualization of healthy direction of flow in meridians, one at a time.

Donna Eden's book on meridian tracing is unfortunately titled *Energy Medicine*. 40 videos on Youtube last time I looked. Classes here http://innersource.net/em

For methods above, pictures of the separate meridians will benefit you unless you have the meridians memorized already. images.Google.com can get you pictures.

Most useful meridian chart I'm aware of

12 Meridian & Five Element Reference Guide

http://www.reflexologyusa.com/html/Online_Store.php

The rest of visualizing a meridian flowing in its healthy direction is how much you enjoy and feel results from visualizing what you wish more of.

View the disturbed meridian, start to end; picture the direction it runs. Imagine this happening in your body. Ask the Light to do TWO things.

1) Ask the Light to clear the UNDERcharge in the meridian. Imagine the Light flowing up and down the meridian until it's balanced.

2) Ask the Light to clear the OVERcharge in the meridian. Imagine the Light flowing up and down the meridian until it's balanced.

3) Go to the next meridian in need of clearing.

4) The next day, try balancing them again. Do this daily until meridians of concern stay in balance.

Notice all the shifts in your interior energy. The more you can feel your inner shifts, the more effective your balance will be.

Using this manual - Two case studies

Use this manual to "connect the dots" between issues and illnesses in yourself and clients.

Example 1: Today a client asked me about a problem with overly frequent urination. I knew from several sessions with her that she is diabetic. My guess was another cause needed to be explored as a primary and causative factor of what she wishes to clear.

I ask a few questions. Meridians come up to be looked at. A water meridian, bladder or kidney, don't you think? I find problems with the physical bladder usually track back to the bladder meridian Not in this case. It tests as tracking back to the kidney meridian.

So I got out my copy of this book. No chart, textbook or manual I know of has as complete an inventory of the psychological aspects and metaphors listed in this book. If you know of a better book, please tell me!

Anyway I got out this resource, looked up KIDNEY Meridian. It offers me a choice: undercharge or overcharge? I test the client: overcharge.

I read her the expressions of overcharged Kidney dysfunction They fit the client's father. We test and they also fit the client's expression in a prior existence.

Before we move to solutions, I test my guess against this client's Highest Guidance: how relevant is Kidney overcharge expressions to her frequent urination? How much of the causative factors have I identified, as seen from her own Higher Guidance?

The response is 60%. Perhaps it benefits us to make a Pie Chart Graph of this disturbance. Because a 60% fraction is larger than 50%, there can be no factor larger than 60% of the problem. This tests as the primary causative factor for this client's body at this time. Lower G.I. tract issues are very frequently connected to negativity from prior existences.

The manual has served its purpose; we have connected the dots between her illness and her issues.

Moving to solutions

Once her disturbance has been looked at from several directions, and there is nothing more major to be uncovered, we move to solutions, to release the stuck negativity interfering with the healthy function of her urinary tract.

She chooses to use self-forgiveness. The client has worked with me many times and knows this routine. For specifics, see Forgive from Your Soul, Slow-Motion Forgiveness booklet. This is the most common solution to release stuck negativity because, Forgiveness is the analogue to subtracting in first grade math.

The client and I work together to compose a few 'forgiveness formulas' to name the negativity she wishes to release. She does the process on three overcharged Kidney expressions. As she facilitates her own process of self-forgiveness, we both feel a lot of trapped "heat" release from her lower left side of her body, a common phenomena when unnecessary overcharge releases.

I test to see if there are additional Kidney overcharge expressions she could usefully clear up. There are. Rather than take up the client's paid time with me and to empower her as a self-healer, I email the client the full text of the overcharged Kidney meridian portion of the manual.

I suggest she experiment with making up and voicing Forgiveness Formulas for other additional over- and undercharged kidney meridian expressions.

Clearing the unconscious almost always has elements of trial and error. This is one meaning of the metaphor of the labyrinth: to navigate the unconscious, there will always be trial and error. This is why in movies analogous to Theseus in the Labyrinth, looking for the Minotaur, he never finds it immediately; he does not find Minotaur in the first place he looks. Why? Because our child within knows an accurate fairy archetype has to include the process of search, trial and error.

"Trial and error" is also called "improvise." To shift stuck energy "out of hiding" and into the Light, we "make stuff up;" as they say in USM, and see if it works. There is no cost for failure. You simply try another experiment until you stumble upon something workable.

Case study 2

I myself had a sharp moderate pain on the back of my right elbow I could not track down to any physical cause. I was in a session as a client with Mimi Castellanos, a gifted Medical Intuitive (HealthyEnergetics.net). She asked herself the question, "Is the pain on any meridian?" Turns out it is on a famous Triple Warmer point, TW 10 with secondary involvement with Small Intestine 8, both points on the back of the elbow.

This insight led to a six weeks of work de-escalating trauma from the amygdala, right jaw nerve etc, all of which tracked back to trauma and PTSD in prior existences, a great example of how pain is our friend in balancing energy.

Q: Do you need to use Bruce's methods to move energy?

A: Not at all. Use whatever self-healing method you have chosen to practice from the Skill Ladder of Self-connection and Energy Medicine: EFT, Immunics, meridian tracing, Touch for Health, etc.

When moving invisible energies is foreground, I encourage you to ask for the Light of the Highest God and Greatest Loving each time. Set you intention at the beginning for your Beloved to be present, to fill, surround, protect and guide you in your session.

Clearing thoroly means, at the end of sessions, clear yourself, clear any second person present. You can ask for the Christ to clear the eight corners of the session room. What's your Energetic Hygiene routine?

Balanced meridian expressions & behaviors

CONCEPTION VESSEL (Also called Central Meridian) ~ No element YIN

Healthy, positive, balanced: I feel good about me the way I am (no deficit of self-esteem).

GOVERNING VESSEL ~ No element YANG

Healthy, positive, balanced: Self-confidence, self-assured stance in life, connected with own personal power without any need to flaunt it, exploit it or boast about it, comfortable standing tall in your own column of Light.

PERICARDIUM (Circulation sex)

Healthy, positive, balanced: On the left, Gratitude for your needs which have been met. On the right, Generosity for what you can give, contribute and make happen next. Aware of needs and opportunities in the present. Enthusiasm, healthy impulse control, healthy interest in the outer world. On the left, satiated, tranquil. On the right, playful risk taking, rejuvenating power of play

TRIPLE WARNER (Triple Heater)

Healthy, positive, balanced: Emotional buoyancy, contented singing, elation, lifting up, living lightly on the Earth, healthy "unbearable lightness of being."

GALL BLADDER

Healthy, positive, balanced: Absence of vengefullness, absence of personal criticisms of specific others. Patience & tolerance towards others, focus on how others can support you accomplishing your own plans. Openness to other's point of view, works well with others. Forbearance, thoughtful choosing. Able to make plans and follow thru on them (Rita Louise). Defusing conflict & useless polarity, healthy assertion of own views, mental flexibility.

LIVER

Healthy teenage enthusiasm. Inspirational youthful vitality and resilience. Shouting for joy, joy bubbling up especially in children and teens. Polite self-assertiveness. Self-motivation, will to become response-able. Trusting. Understanding. Composed socially. Emotionally composed, poise, conscientious, reliable. Flexible to personal changes. Unsuspicious of hostility from others, ready to forgive & forget difficulties. Orderly rhythm between energy and matter.

LUNG

Healthy discernment, intellect at its best. Healthy morality: honesty, humility, mentally accessible. "Humility" captures only some of this; "healthy discrimination" is much closer.

LARGE INTESTINE

Healthy process of what is worth holding onto and what to jettison as used up. Letting go of habits not working for us. Hold onto habits which are working for us. Knowing how long to hold on. Knowing when to let go of anything no longer working for you PACMES. Mentally permeable.

STOMACH

Life tastes good to me now. Healthy taste for healthy resources. Pleased with self. Balancing internal deficits with external nourishments. Smooth sensing of internal conditions and identifying external sources of nourishment. Sensitivity (taste) to emotional disturbance in self and others. Healthy sympathy & liking (deep compassion is more Heart).

Feeling satisfied here in 3D, material contentment and tranquility, Healthy faith & expectancy of good things coming (like a dog waiting expectantly, patiently for a treat).

Adequate & sufficient taste for own creature comforts, healthy taste for the creature comfort of others.

SPLEEN-PANCREAS

Full of the sweet nectar of life, "I've got so much honey, even the bees envy me" (*Whisenant* 220). Awareness of your needs and awareness of what you are doing to get your needs met; therefore, faith and confidence in the future. Harmony, peace-making. Ability to resonate with others and get them to resonate with us, 'resonates well with others.'

Nurturing warmth, accepting, open about feelings. Appropriate consideration of others. Balanced interest in and connection to others.

Healthy playing of roles in life. Creates and manages beneficial roles in life are useful and beneficial to self, family and others; therefore, faith and confidence in one's future.

Healthy sympathy: "I like you. Let's be friends." Many children, especially age four and five, do this with other children near their age (resonating). Singing and children's songs.

HEART MUSCLE

Generous to self and others, personal contentedness. Meeting life's challenges resiliently, not exhausting self. Loving, forgiveness. If all internal organs are adequately and sufficiently connected to the heart; then, content in your personal domain.

Flowing with what can and cannot be controlled towards mutual wellness, i.e., how young King Arthur builds Camelot.

Matching thoughts with feelings; and, feelings with thoughts--easily; therefore, inwardly secure. Alignment of feeling and thinking mind; therefore, capacity for gratefulness, forgiveness, benevolence, compassion, community-building. "I love you," aligned passion, conviction, loyalty to one's own joy without being egocentric.

SMALL INTESTINE

Smooth-flowing assimilation of external resources for building inner coherency and strength. Tolerates solitary activity patiently. Clear of distracting internal confusions. Balanced attention to detail, able to see how small details fit into larger picture, easy travel between details and the large vision. Unconsciously contented; therefore, confidence, emotional endurance, physical vitality.

BLADDER

Healthy alertness, with-it-ness, open alert focus, healthy caution. Natural courage, resolve about what to do. Realistic self-concept. Easy to stand stand up for yourself and face consequences of what you have set in motion. Water easily moving between natural phases of fluidity and ice. Moving between spontaneity and hardness of purpose, as free as the wind and as solid as a rock.

KIDNEY

Trust. Willingness. Calm, steady forward movement, not arrogant or pushy or driven. Inwardly resourceful. Healthy involvement, engagement, neither clinging nor condemning. "Before enlightenment one chops wood and carries water. After enlightenment one chops wood and carries water [willingly]" (koan quoted by *Whisenant* pg. 277). In sexual congress, trusting self; being responsible; unconsciously confident.

A Waldorf-methods approach to learning meridians

Summary ~ A Waldorf-methods approach to learning acupuncture meridians encourages exposing learners to the polarities and patterns evident.

Going further, a whole-brained methods approach to learning acupuncture meridians encourages exposing learners to do two things:

- Memorizing names and placement (L-brain); and

- Direct experience of meridian flows (R-brain).

Research with Mr. Google in 2017 suggests student training methods for learning acupuncture meridians are rarely holistic or whole-brained. Left-brain-only learning predominates to an astonishing degree: learning names and physical placement.

Online-only research suggests existing student training methods for learning acupuncture meridians are out of balance, using only left brain intelligences. Online-only research suggests extreme outer-orientation of meridian learning is even more pronounced in Asian acupuncture literature than in Western schools. Asian TCM student training methods emphasize brute-force memorization (making clear inner mental pictures). Hands-on clinical practice seems intended to augment brute-force memorization.

Hopefully live student classes are more interactive, hands-on and experiential. Hopefully, students are encouraged to feel flow in their own meridians; and then, in clients.

Towards a better balance of training methods, a Waldorf-methods and whole-brain approach to the Inner Dashboard of the 14 major flows in our etheric body is now in view.

Both memorization and clinical experience are necessary. Let's also consider what's missing, by holistic-humanistic criteria.

Western training in Chinese meridians began in the early 1970s at UCLA. The impression is left brain learning methods were paramount.

Starting in 1974 with *Touch for Health, 1st Ed*; and then, Donna Eden's Meridian Tracing (InnerSource.net), a more balanced, holistic-humanistic, left~right brain approach to learning and healing meridians became available. Among other goals, holistic-humanistic students were encouraged to attend to, and expand on, their subjective feeling experience of meridian flows.

In living meridians, the feeling quality of flow is colored by:

- Whether energy is flowing in healthy direction of flow--or not,

- Perceiving a different quality when energy flows backwards against its healthy direction of flow,

- Perceiving stuck energy, uncertain, undecided, which direction to flow,

- Perceiving different qualities in each bilateral meridians of a pair, subjective (inner) percepts of flow, color, taste, smell, sound.

- Differing elemental quality (if perceptible).

A whole-brained, left~right brain grasp of meridians, in a humanistic-holistic framework, includes:

- Memorization of names and placement,

- Encouraging direct experience of flow in meridians.

Whole-brained approach to learning meridians

As a trained Waldorf teacher and Energy Medicine practitioner, I'm aware a Waldorf-methods approach to learning meridians exists.

A Waldorf approach appears to be simpler, clearer and more conducive to whole-brain practice.

In Grade One, the whole of mathematics and number is reduced to polarities, patterns and characters. One example, the abstract idea of odd and even numbers is presented as Boy and Girl numbers, using kids in the class to alternate and demonstrate this.

The whole of drawing is reduced to a polarity of straight and curved in Nature and architecture.

In Grade Five and later, history and biography are made more vivid and impressive by emphasizing polar opposite expressions, even in the same person.

Waldorf teaching methods for any new topic suggest starting with the most obvious, largest polarity; progress to smaller nuances as students can grasp additional finer details.

Many readers will recognize this as "whole-to-part" thinking--this is part of the method. The rest is "not to define but to characterize" (Steiner paraphrase). "Naming" and "Definition" are left brain exercises proclaiming and affirming placement and proximity to other ideas.

"Characterization" is a right brain exercise, related to first impressions, caricature, representation (including parody) and gut instincts. Do both. For audiences younger than puberty, Characterization will be preferred over Definition. For audiences after puberty, the reverse. If you want whole-brain thinkers, after puberty--DO BOTH.

Q: What about Characterizing meridians by their elemental quality?

A: All well and good. However please notice left brain's tendency to use elemental association as a tool for mere PLACEMENT in an abstract TCM scheme of elemental dynamics. Only very few people can directly experience inside themselves, the transformations of five element flow. I believe feeling-sensing the elemental quality directly is a far advanced skill, which few ever master, short of those already highly clairvoyant.

What more students can do is be encouraged to PERCEIVE FLOWS, in their own meridians, whichever sensory channel is most-open for them.

Apart from direct clairvoyance, several polarities and patterns are perceptible in acupuncture meridians. Here's one way to sequence instruction. First:

Origin of the term "meridian" in acupuncture

> The term "meridian" was introduced by Soulie de Morant as the translation for the Chinese word "luo." Yet a more accurate description would be "vessels," "pathways" or "channels," and these terms are sometimes used interchangeably. "Meridian" is typically used to describe the invisible longitudinal lines of the earth, while "vessels" are pathways through which vital substances flow throughout the body.

> http://www.yogiapproved.com/health-wellness/qi-meridians-yin-yang-depth-look-acupuncture/

Second, leave aside Governing Vessel and Conception Vessel. These are much deeper than the 12 more superficial meridians. The two are easy to treat as a pair. Use these to go deeper after students have a feel for the realm of the 12.

Overall front~back pattern of flow

Third: If you had to make a wet-on-wet watercolor painting of the meridians (hint-hint), using red for upflow and blue for downflow, how would you paint?

Please do honor student guesses about representing the polarity of red-upflow and blue-downflow in their paintings. No wrong way to approximate this. The only way to wrongly approximate this is to paint nothing at all.

Afterwards, after class review of student work, lead them to consider these possibilities:

- On the front of the trunk, minus the arms, the main direction is upwards (Stomach meridian in only major meridian going down on front of trunk. Conception also flows up).

- On the sides, Gall Bladder is altogether a downward flow on entire side of the body, both sides (no contradicting meridians whatsoever among the 12).

- On the back, the major direction is down (Back of the body below shoulders "belongs" to Bladder Meridian. Upward flow is represented by the Governing Vessel. Leaving it aside for the moment).

- Our head altogether resists such simple ideas. My suggestion is the cowl shape, like in the Assassin's Creed game and movie. Up to you if it's red or blue. I dunno.

Then have them do a second painting.

Pattern of flow, front and back of limbs

On our inner arms, in anatomical position, facing front, three yin meridians flow down our inner arm (Lng. Pericard. Hrt.)

On our outer arms, in anatomical position, back towards us, three YANG meridians flow up (Lg.Int. Triple. Sm.Int.

On our inner leg, three yin meridians flow up (Kid. Liv. Spl.)

On outside of leg, GB meridian (YANG) flows down, Stomach (YANG) is right on top of Femur and Tibia as they face forward.

The above highlights inner and outer pattern of limbs when learning meridian placement and direction of flow.

On the arms, yin meridians flow down the inner arm; YANG meridians flow up the outer arm.

On our legs, three YANG meridians all travel down (Stom. GB. Bladder); three yin meridians travel up (Spl. Liv, Kid.).

Above section simplified from several references, mostly: http://www.shen-nong.com/eng/principles/distributionmeridians.html › Home › Basic Principles › The Twelve Meridians

Pattern: Meridians flowing between Heaven and Earth

On our inner arms, three yin meridians flow DOWN from Heaven to Earth (Lng. Pericard. Hrt.) Can you perceive a gentle downward spiral?

On our outer arms, three YANG meridians flow from Earth up to Heaven (Lg.Int. Triple. Sm.Int.) Can you perceive a gentle upward spiral?

On our inner leg, three yin meridians flow UP from Earth to Heaven (Kid. Liv. Spl.) Can you perceive a gentle upward spiral?

On the outside of our leg, YANG GB meridian flows down from Heaven to Earth, YANG Stomach is right on top of Femur and Tibia as they face forward. Can you perceive a gentle downward spiral?

I vote for keeping each meridian, its *yin* or YANG quality and direction of flow "embedded" in the inner~outer sides of limbs and front~back sides of torso.

Keeping meridians "embedded" in this manner counteracts the mental tendency to run away and escape form feeling them and into various abstracts tables of meridians and qualities so common in texts. Keeping each meridian associated with a body part is towards feeling its flow. Nomenclature and placement in terminology is half the story; yet, ultimately these will be secondary after ten years of practice. The endgame is knowing the terms AND feeling them in your body and the body of clients.

Guess what? Students will come to their own inner pictures and conceptions for upward-flowing meridians on the inner side of limbs and for downward-flowing meridians on the outer side of limbs. Ask them to speak out their understanding to each other in dyads. Then ask them to write out their understanding on paper.

To Learn More

See the section on Conception-Governing Vessels earlier in this book!

For those interested, behind the four elements, is the pattern of etheric formative forces, discussed most clearly in Man or Matter, 3rd Ed. (1985).

About the Author

Find Health Intuitive Bruce Dickson at https://holisticbrainbalance.wordpress.com

20 videos here: http://www.youtube.com/watch?v=igrhezqeglg

HealingToolbox@gmail.com

InnerSunshine Book Covers and Descriptions

Resources for those looking for self-healing thru self-connection.

All titles dedicated to expanding the ministry of John-Roger.

Caution ~ Some titles and many exercises require facility with self-testing

Most of the booklets and covers. All books available in eBOOK, most available in paper. All written in an interactive, FUN style by a practicing Health Intuitive with training from Waldorf teacher training MSIA, USM, NVC; and, study of IFS.

Best Practice in Group Process Series

Heartfelt Facilitators Notebook; Best Practices Facilitating Large/Small Group Events (2022)

To my knowledge, the first user-friendly book on the WHAT, WHY, HOW and TIPS for facilitating live group events, with a heartfelt look and feel.

Intended audience for this project is:

- working facilitators, male and female

- facilitators-in-training, and

- anyone interested in live group facilitating.

The author believes women naturally have more strengths for most live facilitating, than most men. Male facilitators benefit from internalizing the heartfelt ethic and feminine values of connecting, cooperating, collaborating and negotiating.

Some topics here pertain to live-streamed virtual events, other topics less so. Feel free to skip around per your interests. Scripts also available.

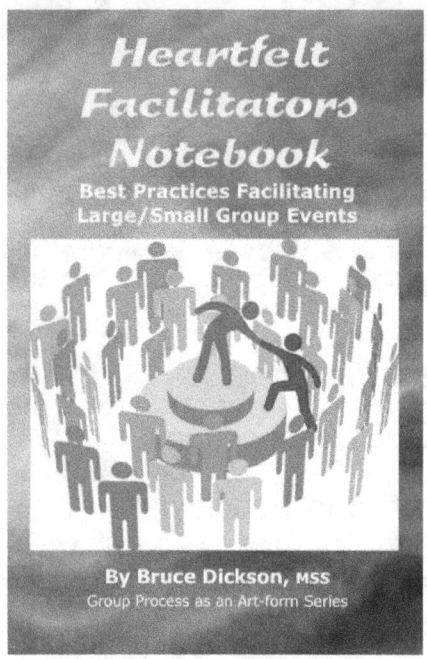

Milling and Dyad Questions for Learning Conversations in Personal Growth Live Events

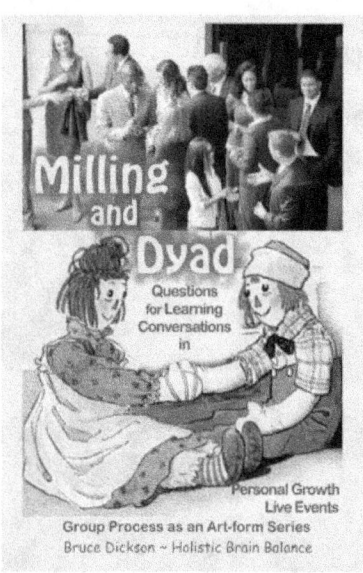

Scripted Closed-Eye-Processes for Live Personal Growth Event Facilitators and Group Leaders

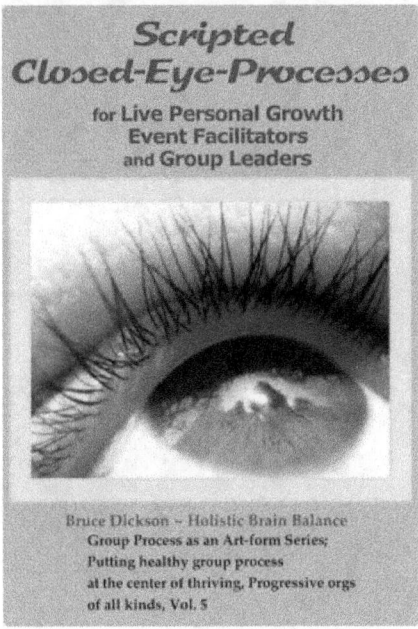

New Directions in Holistic Brain Balance

New, shorter booklets

Description of contents for each book at
https://HolisticBrainBalance.wordpress.com

1) **Holistic Neurology;** Connecting with Our Two Nervous Systems, Head-brain and Gut-Brain - Our Two Nervous Systems, Head-spine (cerebral) and enteric (gut), Neurology for purposes of personal growth, the physiological basis for Self-esteem and Self-concept (2nd ed 2023)

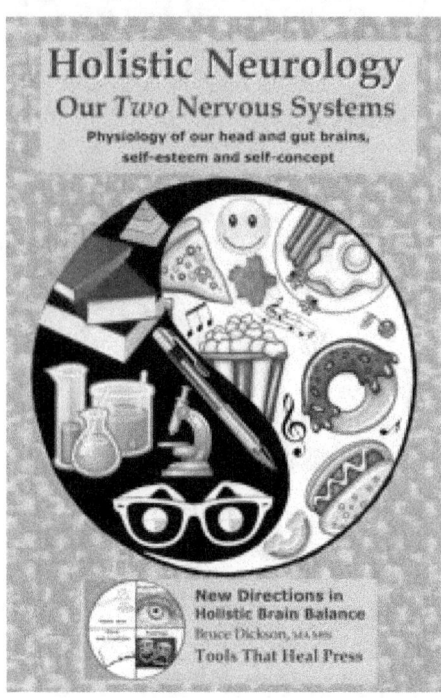

2) **Our Four Brain Quadrants**, New Directions in Holistic Brain Balance (Holistic Brain Balance Vol 2)

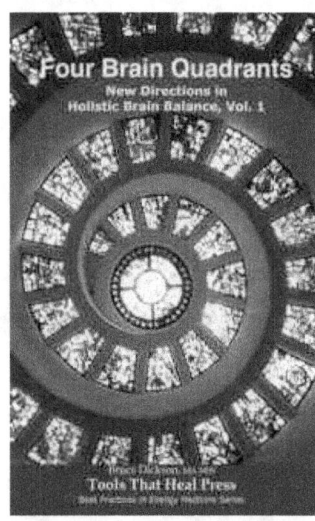

Reactivity Is Our Best Friend, New Directions in Holistic Brain Balance (Vol 3)

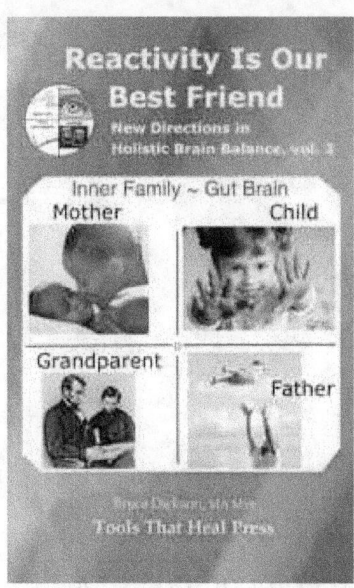

Forgive from Your Soul, Slow-Motion Self-Forgiveness, the Missing Manual (99 cents) (Holistic Brain Balance Vol 4)

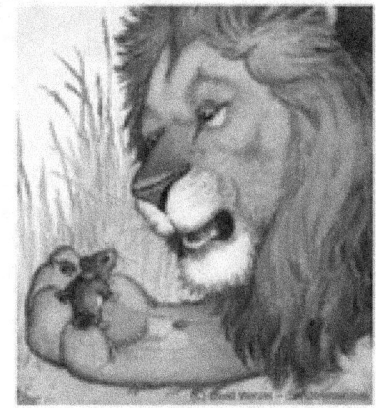

Inner Sunshine, How to Make More of It; Assessing Neurotransmitter Production with Self-testing; The simple complexity of our unconscious (Holistic Brain Balance Vol 5)

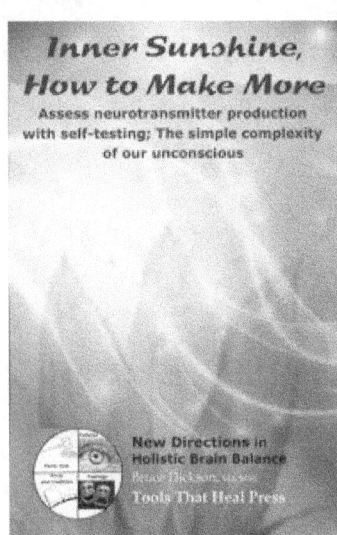

Balance on All Levels PACME+Soul; *Finally, a general holistic experimental method; The Three Sciences we use everyday; Holistic Psychology 2.0.* Also being released as chapters. Some chapters up now as eBook.

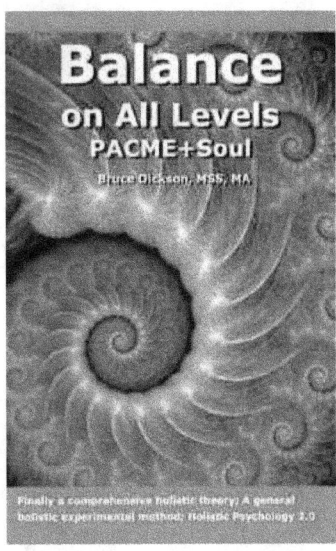

In the 1900s, psychology focused on only three human intelligences: physical, mental, emotional. A three-legged chair, three legs makes a stool stable. This worked as a partial model of waking human psyches--in the 1900s.

Differentiating multiple human intelligences had to wait for John Gardner's Multiple Intelligences (1983). Since 2000, given several decades of Energy Medicine innovation and experiment, many intuit; and some can perceive, multiple intelligences all the way down in our unconscious, to the cell and sometimes DNA level. We have many more intelligences active in our waking psyche than most people even dream of.

Not everyone is ready for four, eight, or 12 active intelligences. Feeling overwhelmed? I call this the problem of Our Many Selves. If you can't learn about your many selves with acceptance and love, stay out of the kitchen. My guess is many Cultural Creatives are ready for an expanded reframing of our psyche and for keys to balance on all levels. If that's you, read on.

The more we understand, ground and purify our multiple intelligences, the richer human experience is for us individually.

Imagine soul in the human experience as a balancing act, balancing between excess and deficient, on many levels at once. Our balance as a soul in the human experience plays out in how we respond to life; either with, conditioned habits--or choosing a new way to respond (free choice).

Surprisingly, 5% of free choice in our waking psyche is capable of balancing the 95% of our psyche which is conditioned habits.

99 cent eBooks

You have FIVE bodies, PACME, Spiritual Geography 101

Reversal of Learning Style at Puberty; How Developing Self-esteem

Precedes SElf-concept--and Why; Self-confidence Equals Self-esteem

Plus Self-concept

Breast Cancer & Over-giving; Therapeutic Metaphors for Women's Issues

From Five Animal Senses to 12 or More Human Senses

Forgive from Your Soul, Slow Motion Forgiveness, the Missing Manual

How We Heal; and, Why do we get sick? Including 35 more precise Q&A on wellness.

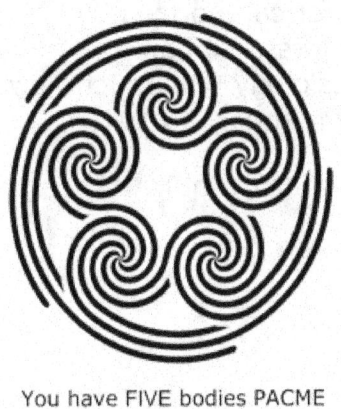

You have FIVE bodies PACME
Spiritual Geography 101

Bruce Dickson, MSS, MA

Tools That Heal Press
Best Practices in Self-Healing System Series
HealingToolbox.org

A fundamental distinction John-Roger and others make early and often is the useful tool of Spiritual Geography, discerning we have not one body here on Earth, but FIVE. Take away or compromise with any one of these bodies and we become less than fully human, less than fully capable of giving and receiving love.

Best Practices in Energy Medicine Series

The two best sellers:

Meridian Metaphors, Psychology of the meridians and major organs

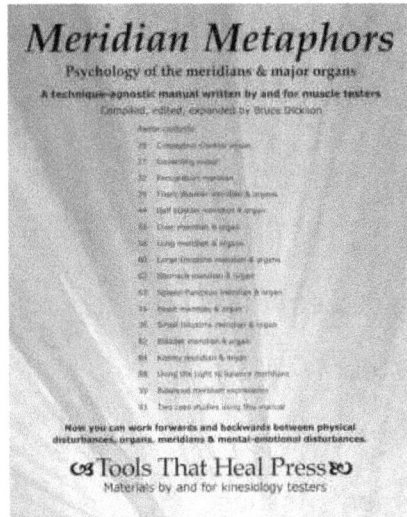

Ever wonder what the connection between meridians, organs and emotions is? Ever think TCM had a start on good ideas but much was missing?

Now anyone can work either forwards or backwards, between disturbed organs and meridians on one hand; and, disturbed mental-emotional states on the other hand.

All descriptions begin with healthy function. Disturbances are further categorized by under- and overcharge conditions. Includes the myths and metaphors of under-overcharged organs-meridians condensed from Psychological Kinesiology plus much new material from other clinical practitioners. 22,000 words 100 page manual, 8 x10"

NEW Energy Anatomy; Nine new views of the human being that don't require clairvoyance

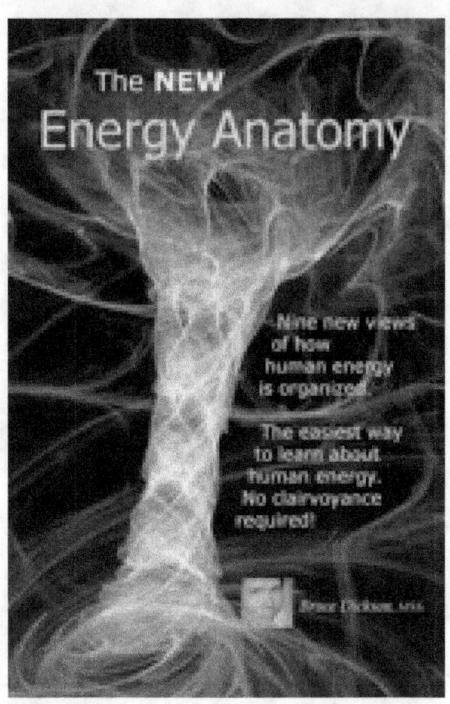

An easier, simpler, faster way to learn about human energy system compared to the chakra system. The NEW Energy Anatomy is a better entry point for students to developing sensitivity. Each view is testable with kinesiology of any and all kinds. You be the judge!

Particularly useful for energy school students and sensitive persons using testing to sort out their abundant perceptions. More generally useful for efforts to become more Coherent, Integrated and Aligned (the new CIA). Coupled with Touch for Health, EFT, Energy Medicine or PTS Masters and Doctorate programs, these views facilitate making your aura brighter.

Human energy is organized:

1) RIGHT~*left* in the body, YANG~*yin* in the body, from the neck down.

2) Top and bottom, enteric and cerebral nervous systems, Holistic Neurology.

3) Front and back, CV-GV, Think Clark Kent~Superman.

4) As four zones of laughter Hee-hee, Ha-ha, heh-heh, Ho-ho.

5) Top and bottom in our gut brain, divided top and bottom, feeling above (heh, hed and willingness below (Ho, ho).

6) Four quadrants in our gut brain, an Inner Family.

7) Four quadrants in our head, an Inner Court.

8) The back of our head is willingness to heal our past.

9) Hip stability is a Ring of Loving you can strengthen.

Other material includes the Law of Gentleness for healers, coaches and counselors.

40,800 words 245 p. in 6x9 format.

1 Your Habit Body; An Owner's Manual; Gut-brain Axis 2.0

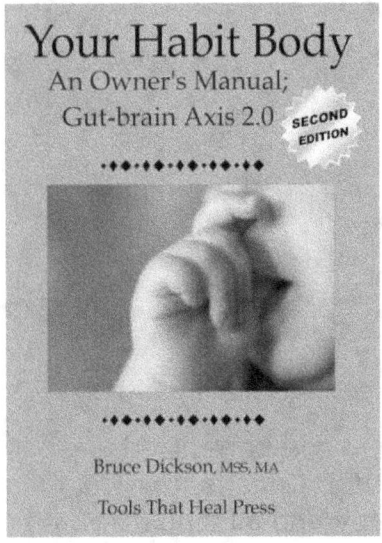

Second edition of Your Habit Body; An Owner's Manual

A habit is one or more learned behaviors, conditioned to repeat. Habits are formed by repetition. Habits are strengthened by repetition. Why do we allow and promote forming habits? Our unconscious stores them so they can be played back when useful. Playing back an old habit pattern takes less energy than focusing to come up with a completely new unscripted behavior response.

In this way, each person's collection of stored habits available for replay, is analogous to an old honky-tonk jukebox, playing 45 RPM single records. You can choose which habit you wish to play; or, if set on automatic, it plays back the most popular tunes. This is our Habit Body at work.

1 Personal Habit Tracking as a Spiritual Exercise (2021)

Increase Self-connection; Build a Bridge to Your Inner Wisdom

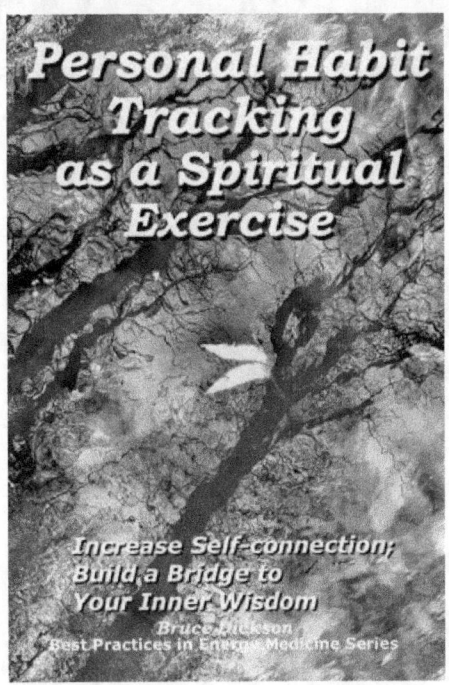

Personal Habit Tracking as a Spiritual Exercise

Increase Self-connection;
Build a Bridge to
Your Inner Wisdom
Bruce Dickson
Best Practices in Energy Medicine Series

YOU are the greatest mystery worth solving. Tracking, experiential and hands-on, is a Best Practice in self-connection, self-healing and self-befriending. Do you need a friend? This could be it.

What do you need to do a tracking experiment? You need:

- A question you have high interest in getting a second opinion on,

- Curiosity about your habits, your own Habit Body. What am I doing? What is working for

me? what is NOT workable for me? This facilitates self-healing on all levels,

- A clear idea of who you are asking, which internal part. A simple, workable model of your psyche, is needed here.

- A format in which your inner response yesterday can be compared to your inner response today can be compared.

This book alternates between practical tracking topics; and, sketching out contexts useful for you to have a clear conceiving of what you are doing in your own tracking experiments.

1 You are a Hologram Becoming Visible to Your Self

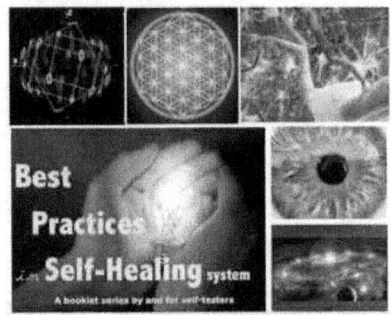

You are a
Hologram
Becoming visible
to your self

Best Practices in **Self-Healing** system
A booklet series by and for self-testers

Bruce Dickson ~ HealingToolbox.org

The bigger part of us, our inner child, immune system, high self, "true self," "divine connection"--however you term it, is invisible to us for several reasons--but you can change this and get to know the "bigger you."

The metaphor of a hologram is a good way to see the "bigger you" behind all the familiar smokescreens.

A hologram metaphor assists us to reframe the "bigger you" with new eyes. As modern people, we understand a hologram has both three dimensions and internal structure. These are useful metaphors for our inner dimensions and the structures in our sub- and unconscious. Our psyche is a hologram of physical, imaginal, emotional, mental and mythological potentials. Some are fully activated, many are not. Some are stuck and dysfunctional.

What we have inside us can be understood in terms of a 3D framework and a hologram is the way to "see" this, the structure of the "bigger you."

A full discussion of how the "bigger you" is structured and organized as a hologram, and the history of this idea, in included in this work.

Self-Healing 101! 2nd ed.

Seven Experiments in Self-healing You Can Do at Home to Awaken the Inner Healer

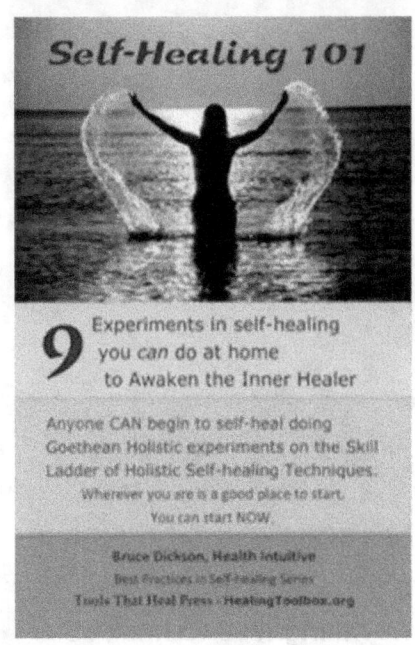

Anyone CAN self-heal. Wherever you are is a good place to start. You can start NOW

For those looking to go deeper into self-healing and/or begin or deepen their practice of self-muscle-testing. Alternatively, for those teaching others how to self-muscle-test.

Self-healing and self-muscle-testing is outside the exhausted residue of Cartesian-Newtonian Science. Self-healing and self-muscle-testing is really part of the more appropriate newer Goethean Holistic Science; that is, all results, all phenomena, are replicable but NOT by all persons, at all places and all times, regardless of intention. Rather results are replicable primarily in the domain of one person.

Q: How do I begin our own journey of self-healing in the domain of one person, myself?

A: We move to a more experiential approach to self-healing beginning with

- Self-acceptance, self-love

- prayers of self-protection

- self-sensitivity

- self-permission to make testing experiments.

In hands-on Goethean Holistic Science experiments, there is no penalty for failure, none at all--as long--as you learn something from every experiment.

The only wrong way to experiment is not to try at all (John-Roger).

Willingness to heal is the pre-requisite for all healing

This quote from Bertrand Babinet begins exploration and expansion of some of Bertrand Babinet's wonderful legacy of theory and method.

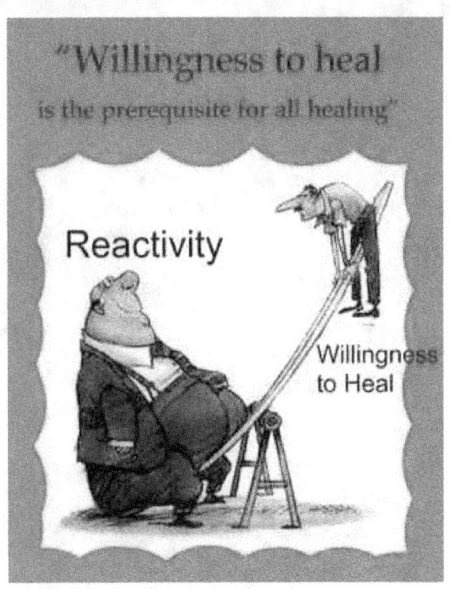

"Willingness to heal is the prerequisite for all healing"

Reactivity

Willingness to Heal

If you can do testing by any method, you can measure your own willingness to heal. Self-testers can measure their own willingness to heal, in your inner child.

This tells you if your silent partner is ready to heal what you wish to heal. You can use this to explore where you are most ready to grow.

Have clients? The effectiveness of any energetic session can be estimated AHEAD OF TIME, with surprising accuracy--before you begin working! Practitioners in any and all modalities, are encouraged measure willingness to heal FIRST!

Save your self from wasting effort when clients are of two minds on their issue and do not know this. The higher the number on a scale of 1-10, the more momentum your client has to heal on that issue.

Willingness to heal is the key to aligning and integrating the three selves. Willingness is where the whole topic of the 3S leads.

NOTE ~ This booklet assumes readers can already either self-test using kinesiology testing—K-testing, dowsing, or some other form; or, can follow instructions to use any partner to do two-person testing, termed Client

Controlled Testing. Problems with your own testing? Don't trust your own results? See the training protocol breakthroughs in Self-Healing 101.

Unconscious Patterns in the Light of the Inner Child and NLP

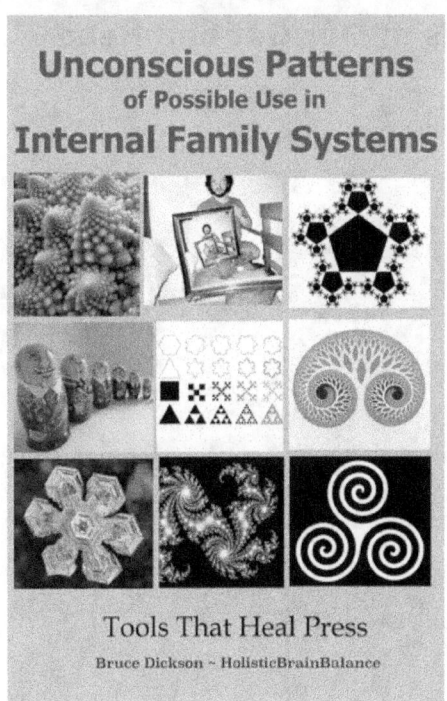

Unconscious Patterns
of Possible Use in
Internal Family Systems

Tools That Heal Press
Bruce Dickson ~ HolisticBrainBalance

What makes us human is primarily invisible. What makes us TRULY human is ALTOGETHER invisible: honesty, compassion, love, willingness to serve our self and others.

Most readers grew up learning our psyche is a locked "black box." We were taught the contents of our psyche are unknown, probably unknowable. Now we know better. Building with NLP, the Inner Child and Energy Medicine methods matured since 1990, many Unconscious Patterns have been uncovered and documented.

The big Aha! for most people is our unconscious is highly patterned and you can understand these patterns. We simply need to play the Blind Detective Game. How much of our psyche is patterning? Up to 95%. Only 5% of us is NOT patterned, the 5% of us where active, deliberate, conscious choice occurs. Soul is choice.

Hundreds, maybe millions of UPs exist. What this book can so is:

- Show Unconscious Patterns are worthwhile, if psychology is your beat,

- Show UPs are worth learning if your purpose is self-healing and/or work with clients,

- Show NLP Metaprograms was Day One of this, only the start,

- Outline some major and minor categories.

The more aware you are of these patterns, the less likely you are to be run by them. The more aware of them, the more likely you are to "be at choice." Soul is choice.

1 Inner Family + Inner Court, The Four Archetypes of Our Gut and Head

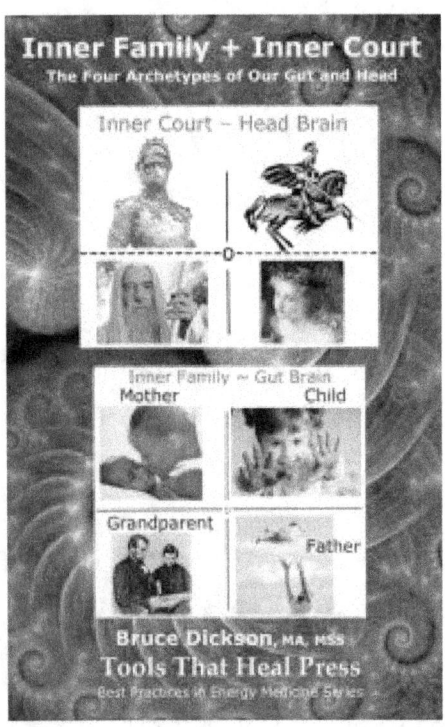

Builds on and expands the work of Paul Dennison, Ned Herrmann, Katherine Benziger and Bertrand Babinet's Babinetics.

We can now bring all these together in the context of ecumenical spirituality, "God is my Partner."

Together all the pieces, give us adequate and sufficient complexity to model our psyche and personality. The ecumenical spirituality piece contributes adequate-sufficient psychic self-protection when dealing with invisible energies.

From Paul we have muscle testing proven as a reliable experimental method--in the domain on one single individual at a time. From Ned and Katherine we have four head quadrants. Bertrand experimented to understand how a similar quadrant architecture existed in or gut brain as well. He was the first to explore quadrants with self-muscle-testing.

Each quadrant connects with an archetype: Inner Mother, Inner Father, Inner Child and Inner Wise-accepting Grandparent. Each archetype stores learned behaviors, values, talents and responses to 3D life. Our four memory archetypes play back recorded habits, to the best of their ability, as appropriate according to their maturity. Which habits you choose to express, when and how--is your uniqueness.

The intelligence of our Habit Body is here. Your Habit Body, An Owner's Manual, is useful preparation for the current volume.

The Five Puberties, a Three Selves Journal on Children

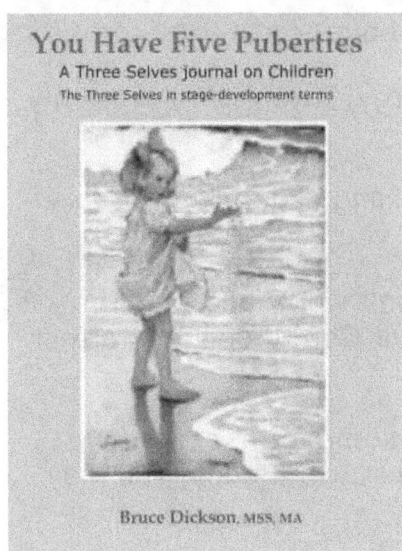

Growing new eyes to see children and stage-development afresh is the goal of this booklet. It builds on the foundation of the other volumes—or--can be read alone. Children are viewed thru lenses not often used: body posture, stories the body tells, animals, plants, the succession of puberties--at least four puberties--each of us undergoes on our journey towards independent thinking.

Finally, we glance at what progress has been made towards a functional typology of children's temperaments in Anthroposophy, MBTI and Katherine Benziger, providing some directions for fruitful further study. The perplexing problem of how children's typology differs from adult typology, is brought close to resolution.

Adequate and Sufficient Psychic Self-protection

For Healers, Sensitives and Energy Medicine Practitioners

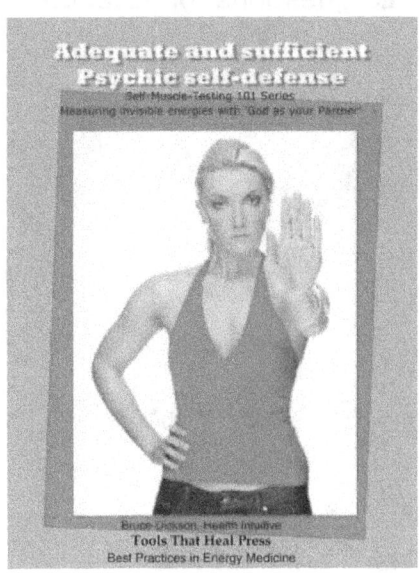

The vast majority of our unresolved disturbances are both *invisible* and *unconscious*.

"Working with energy" is a lay person's way of expressing the above.

I see so many healers and students working *un-safely* with energy, I wanted to share my experience with self-protection in Energy Medicine.

Adequate and sufficient psychic-self-protection is the art of avoiding negativity from getting on you, in you, around you and polluting-contaminating you.

Your intention to be safe and not traffic in negativity counts. Don't worry because worry is an opening to negativity. Simply do the best you can, and ask for God to be your Partner in as many ways as possible.

This booklet is for persons who can already self-muscle-test, in some form, or who are willing to learn. You may use muscles; you may not. You may test with Buddy, you may not.

If you can perform the following self-tests—you are ready for the exercises in this booklet.

If you cannot perform these self-tests, you'll likely have more immediate success looking at the beginning rungs of the Skill Ladder of Energy Medicine Methods; and, with the exercises in *Self-Healing 101, 2nd ed*.

World's easiest questions to self-test on

Note each pair of questions are polar opposites. Overlapping conditions are hopefully absent.

Call in the Light of the Highest God and Greatest Loving, to fill, surround, protect and guide you.

You pass if you get clear responses meaningful to your conscious self, you have at least some confidence in your responses. These are also good practice questions for students learning.

The questions often work best when asked OUT LOUD:

My name is _____. (your real name).

My name is _____. (some other name, i.e., Rumpelstiltskin)

This is my yes. (confirming your signal for "true for me now")

This is my no. (confirming your signal for "not true for me now")

I am in a male body now. (this will be yes or no for you)

I am in a female body now. (this will be yes or no for you)

1 Rudolf Steiner's Fifth Gospel in Story Form

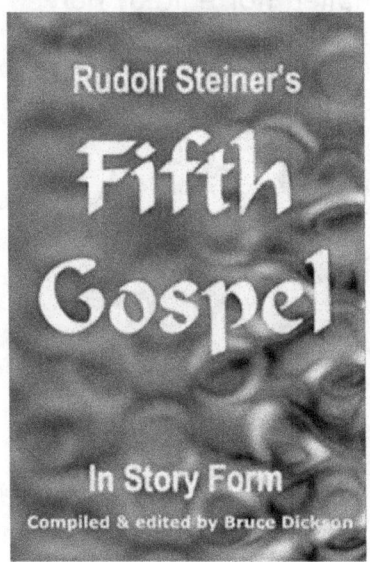

One of the wonderful experiences of my Waldorf teacher training was in a comfy living room, with a group of friends, reading aloud Rudolf Steiner's Fifth Gospel transcripts, round-robin style, a paragraph at a time. We read a chapter each night over the 12 Days of Christmas. If you've done this, maybe you also felt the pull to draw closer to this material. I certainly did.

Dr. Steiner's aim was to update the biography of Jesus of Nazareth, in light of the expanded psychological understanding of karma and reincarnation flourishing in the West between 1880 and 1920.

The imaginative capacity of humankind, our increased ability to process metaphor, demonstrated by Depth Psychology and Carl Jung, made possible this portrait of Jesus of Nazareth and what he transformed into. RS's Fifth Gospel remains the most psychologically astute portrait of Jesus of Nazareth this author is aware of.

An unexpected function of this material is it can support people who have lost the thread of connection with their own internal Christ spark, our immortal-eternal soul. Steiner's Fifth Gospel is an opportunity to pick up the thread of their own connection again. RS's ideas can be very healing to many conventional ideas about Jesus of Nazareth.

What Steiner found in the Akashic Records, regarding the life of Jesus of Nazareth, was a series of "story book images." These are apparently quite closely and faithfully approximated by both children's Sunday School images of the life of Christ; and also by, traditional stained glass windows of the Stations of the Cross.

If you know him, you won't be surprised to hear Steiner dove into and behind these images to penetrate their inner reality; and then, articulate it in modern language for modern minds.

Steiner's verbatim lecture transcripts of his investigations were published in a book called The Fifth Gospel, but his basic clairvoyant research was never compiled nor edited; nor, was any attention paid to building a mood.

The Meaning of Illness is Now an Open Book - Cross-referencing Illness and Issues ($1.85 eBook)

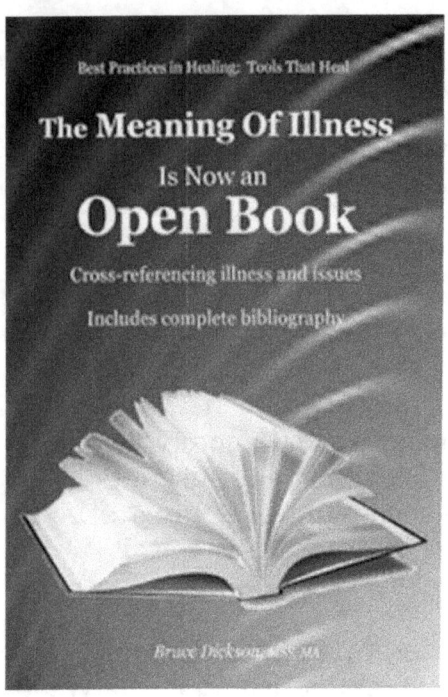

Virtually unknown to the public, EIGHT excellent, peer-reviewed books exist correlating illnesses and mental-emotional issues as of 2013.

It's now possible to simply look up the meaning of physical illnesses, the causative issues behind health concerns. Some combination of these mental-emotional issues is what oppresses your organs, tissues and cells.

For persons with their own Healing Toolbox, they can simply get busy doing what you can to locate, address and resolve these issues. Muscle testing, kinesiology testing of any kind is the most convenient way to navigate to which issue is "live" in you.

If you don't know where your Healing Toolbox is or what's in it, you can always find a Self-Healing Coach, Health Intuitive or Medical Intuitive. Find someone who works with loving.

Those interested in the mental-emotional meaning of illnesses tend to be, self-healers, self-muscle-testers, holistic practitioners, kinesiology practitioners, Medical and Health Intuitives, energy detectives of all kinds and anyone interested in what used to be called "psychosomatic medicine."

Ill-informed, useless and eccentric literature in this field does exist. These are the books I recommend.

Additional material concerns how one Medical Intuitive views his field and his practice:

- Illness as a healing metaphor.

- Willingness to heal is the pre-requisite to heal

- Summary of some very recent protocols and methods for connecting the dots between illnesses and issues.

Chapter Four has some original research on therapeutic metaphors for illness: Cancer and tumors in general, Stroke, SIDS, Autism, Alzheimer's, ADHD, Attention deficit, Hyperactive disorder.

A Proposed Wikipedia page upgrade on "Medical Intuitive"

Shadow Hero Workbook - Lessons to purify the Hero archetype in you; Healthy vs. Unhealthy Hero behavior; Unconscious Patterns 201

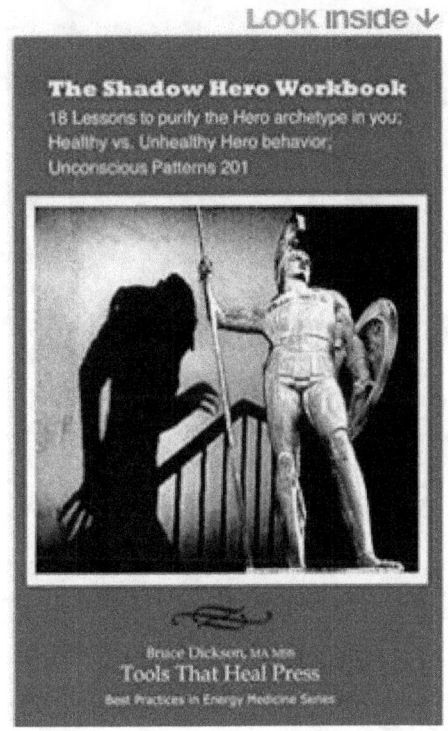

Sooner or later everyone in personal-spiritual growth, purifies their gifts and talents of unwanted Shadow Hero behaviors. Anyone NOT doing this?

Perhaps the first booklet in Hero Archetype literature attempting systematic access to disturbed sub- and unconscious Hero patterns; along with, therapeutic directions for resolving them.

This is NOT my Hero story, NOT a rehash of Campbell's hero cycle. The Workbook is stages of the Hero's cycle re-arranged by psychological category, as possible to do.

18 short lessons designed to increase awareness of dysfunctional Hero patterns. 18 categories of functional and dysfunctional hero behavior are outlined. Therapeutic direction is suggested to clear each, compatible with methods of your own choosing.

All shadow behavior tends to be UNconscious. We're only most conscious of our waking human experience from the neck-up. Still, we're responsible for all habits-expressions in the two lower thirds of our psyche, sub- and unconscious.

Again, self-muscle-testing remains the easiest, cheapest, most direct method to navigate invisible-unconscious issues.

How We Heal; and, Why do we get sick?

Including 35 better, more precise questions on wellness and healing, answered by a Medical Intuitive

Why every illness is a healing metaphor A theory of Cellular Awakening, short version.

Your personal beliefs-myths about healing.

#1: If we understand our problems, they will be healed.

#2: If you don't know and don't understand, then you can't heal.

#3: Personal-spiritual change takes a long time and is always a slow process. After all, you've had the problem for a long time.

#4: If you've had a negative belief for a long time, it will take a long time to change.

#5: If you change quickly, it must be superficial and not long lasting.

#6: I can't change; "This is the way I am; I'll always be this way."

#7: If you are middle-aged or older, it is too late to change.

#8: Changing old behaviors and thought patterns is often difficult and painful, "No pain, no gain."

Why is pain allowed? Why do I put up with so much pain in my body?

Can you help me see disease from Spirit's point of view?

18 more questions addressed.

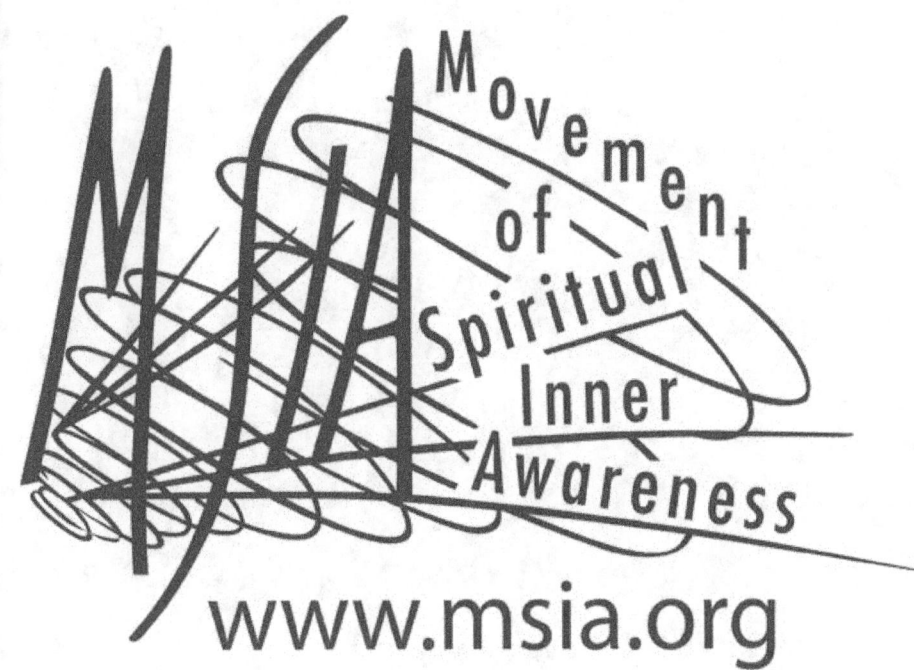

www.msia.org

MSIA Discourses http://www.msia.org/discourses

Forgiveness, Key to the Kingdom, by John-Roger

The Emotion Code, by Bradley Nelson

Messages From the Body, by Michael Lincoln

Touch for Health, 2nd Ed, by Mathew Thie

Changing Lives Through Redecision Therapy, by Goulding & Goulding

Scripts People Live: Transactional Analysis of Life Scripts by Claude Steiner

Core Transformation, by Connierae Andreas

Your Body Speaks Your Mind, 2nd ed. by Deb Shapiro (junior version of Messages from the Body)

> The best solution is always loving
>
> Did you enjoy this? Please share.
>
> If you get stuck, give me a call.

What if a fraction of the new replacement culture, you and I are creating now, will begin around self-healing and training activity as the cultural benefit of the hard work of building new, sustainable, intentional community?

www.ingramcontent.com/pod-product-compliance
Lightning Source LLC
Chambersburg PA
CBHW081130170526
45165CB00008B/2614